Understanding Girls with ADHD

How they feel and why they do what they do

Published by Advantage Books, LLC
8101 Connecticut Avenue
Suite C-406
Chevy Chase, Maryland 20815

First Edition published 1999
Second Edition published 2015

Printed in the United States of America

ISBN 978-0-9714609-7-3

Library of Congress Cataloging-in-Publication Data

Nadeau, Kathleen G.
Understanding Girls with ADHD / Kathleen Nadeau, Ellen Littman, Patricia Quinn — Second Edition
p. cm.

Previous edition published: Advantage Books, 1999.
ISBN 0-9660366-5-4 (paperback)
1. Attention-deficit-disordered children.
2. Girls — Mental health.
3. Hyperactive Children.
I. Littman, Ellen.
II. Quinn, Patricia O.
III. Title.
RJ506.H9N333 1999
618.92'8589'0082 – dc21

Case histories in this book are either composites of several patients' histories or are stories submitted by actual patients or their families. Identities have been changed to protect patient confidentiality.
The term ADHD is used in this book in order to conform to DSM-5 guidelines. It is intended to include all aspects of the disorder, including all subtypes of the disorder.

Cover and interior design, Randy Martin, martinDESIGN.info

10 9 8 7 6 5 4 3 2

Understanding Girls with ADHD

How they feel and why they do what they do

Kathleen G. Nadeau, Ph.D.
Ellen B. Littman, Ph.D.
Patricia O. Quinn, M.D.

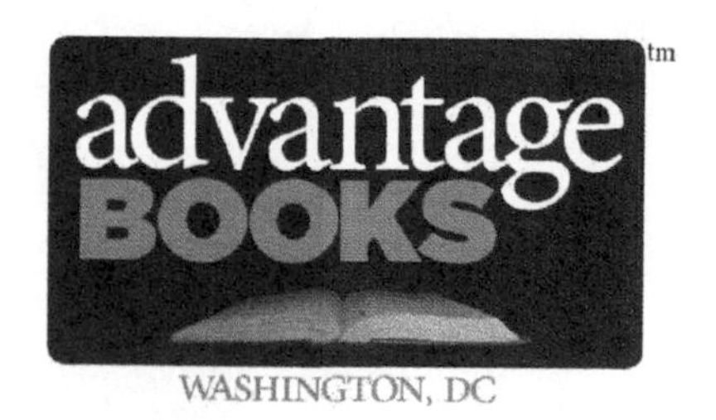

WASHINGTON, DC

DEDICATION

We would like to dedicate this book to all the girls and women that we have known over the years who have taught us to better understand what it is like to be a girl with Attention Deficit Hyperactivity Disorder (ADHD). We have come a long way. But there is much to learn. In partnership with them, we can move forward together, expanding and improving our understanding, making it more likely that future girls with ADHD will grow up to lead authentic, self-affirming lives.

And to the professionals, who have taken up the call to conduct research and thereby increase knowledge and understanding when it comes to girls with ADHD, we thank you.

Kathleen G. Nadeau, Ph.D.
Ellen B. Littman, Ph.D.
Patricia O. Quinn, M.D.

TABLE OF CONTENTS

ABOUT THE AUTHORS

KATHLEEN NADEAU, PH.D. is a clinical psychologist who has specialized in ADHD and related conditions for more than 25 years. During that time, she has written books for children, teens, college students, adults, girls and women with ADHD, always focusing on positive, practical problem-solving. Her focus throughout her career has been to identify under-served ADHD sub-populations and try to increase awareness and services for these populations. In 2000, she received the CHADD Hall of Fame Award for her ground-breaking work on girls and women with ADHD. Dr. Nadeau continues in clinical practice at the Chesapeake ADHD Center of Maryland, in Silver Spring, MD, where she serves as director. Dr. Nadeau continues to write and to lecture both nationally and internationally.

ELLEN LITTMAN, PH.D. is a clinical psychologist who has focused on ADHD and its comorbid issues for more than 27 years. In her private practice just north of New York City, Dr. Littman focuses on a high IQ adult and adolescent ADHD population. She specializes in identifying and treating the often misinterpreted or overlooked presentations of ADHD in girls and women. Her areas of expertise include working with families coping with the far-reaching impact of ADHD, and with those who have experienced early trauma. Educated and trained at Brown, Yale, and Long Island Universities, and the Albert Einstein College of Medicine, she has been described as a pioneer in the field of gender issues in ADHD in the American Psychological Association Monitor. Widely published and quoted, Dr. Littman lectures internationally and provides training to professionals.

PATRICIA QUINN, M.D. is a developmental pediatrician, who has specialized in child development and psychopharmacology for more than 40 years. Her main focus is Attention Deficit Hyperactivity Disorder (ADHD) and on her website (www.addvance.com), she answers important questions about this disorder. For the last two decades, Dr. Quinn has devoted her attention to the issues confronting girls and women with ADHD and feels a strong commitment to helping them to identify and manage issues specific to their gender. In 2000, Dr. Quinn received the CHADD Hall of Fame Award for her work in this area. Dr. Quinn is the author of more than 20 books on ADHD for children, adults, and professionals including the award-winning, *Attention, Girls! A Guide to Learn All About Your ADHD for girls 8-13* and *100 Questions and Answers about ADHD in Women and Girls.*

FOREWORD

IT WAS NOT ALL THAT LONG AGO, in retrospect, that clinicians and scientists alike believed that ADHD existed largely if not exclusively in boys. Despite the surge of information on girls and women with ADHD that currently exists, the history of neglect of females with ADHD is a dispiriting legacy to overcome.

As a graduate student and young investigator in the field back in the 1970s and 1980s, I came to believe myself that the study of ADHD was one and the same as the study of boys and men with ADHD. But I was plagued by the sense that the field's information was incomplete. How could ADHD skip girls altogether? By the early 1990s, the National Institutes of Health had begun to issue guidelines relevant to the study of a wide range of medical diseases and issues in both men and women.[1] For scientific and political reasons, I began to take up the call.

Thus, twenty years ago I prepared a major grant application for the National Institute of Mental Health. In this document my team and I proposed utilizing the summer camp methodologies we had deployed for boys with ADHD[2,3] to investigate a large sample of girls, whom we considered to be grossly under-represented in the existing research literature. Although the field was beginning to believe that girls could experience ADHD, their numbers in scientific papers were small and conclusions fairly speculative. Interest was clearly growing,[4] but there were not the kinds of data on:

a. Girls with ADHD in naturalistic settings (e.g., summer camps), in which information on academic performance, social behavior, cognitive processing, family interactions, and self-perceptions could be synthesized; or

b. Long-term follow-up into adolescence and adulthood with respect to developmental trajectories and lifelong patterns of symptoms, impairments, and resilience.

The grant proposal struck a chord: it received an unprecedentedly strong priority score in 1995. Indeed, the review panel commented on the need, expressed in the application, for not just gender comparison studies (i.e., those directly comparing males and females) but investigations of girls with ADHD in their own right, in the context of all-female contexts. As a result, our team began preparing recruitment of participants for each of three consecutive summer programs, which were held in 1997, 1998, and 1999.

Despite our apprehension that we would not be able find a viable sample, once we had advertised and discussed the planned programs with physicians, mental health centers, a range of clinicians, and schools in the Bay Area, the telephone began to ring off the hook. From more than 1200 inquiries, we applied rigorous selection criteria and, after a multi-gated screening and assessment battery that spanned multiple hours of contact with parents, teachers, and the girls themselves, ended up with a sample of 140 girls with ADHD and an age- and ethnicity-matched comparison sample of 88 girls without ADHD. We began with selection criteria that allowed a wide net but, in the end, insisted that the sample meet full diagnostic criteria for ADHD, the same as exist for males. This all-female, elementary-school-aged sample was ethnically and socio-economically diverse, comprising both the Combined type of ADHD (i.e., girls with high levels of both inattention and impulsivity/hyperactivity) and the Inattentive type of ADHD (i.e., girls with purer inattention and disorganization).

After their participation in our intensive, ecologically valid summer programs, which prioritized multi-informant and multi-method evaluations of as many aspects of their lives as we could feasibly assess, we began publishing findings regarding their behavior and performance across a wide array of domains.[5-12] With these initial publications, we extended the meta-analytic findings of this period that were synthesizing data on existing female samples,[13, 14] demonstrating the clear academic, social, neuropsychological, and family-related deficits of our sample. Along with reports on other female samples,[15] these data portrayed, in stark terms, the high levels of impairment related to female manifestations of ADHD. That is, girls with ADHD suffer in the same ways as do boys, with even greater chances of being rejected by peers and of showing deficits in math and executive functioning.

Prior to the initial programs, I had let all families know that our intention — continued funding willing — was to follow their daughters for the rest of their lives. With additional grant support, we therefore embarked on a prospective follow-up during adolescence[16,17] and, via another grant, a second follow-up during their early years of adulthood.[18] Because of our relentless tracking and monitoring of the sample, because of the close relationships we had formed during the programs, and because of our creative use of social media (e.g., Facebook), we evaluated 92% of the sample at an average age of 14 for our five-year follow-up and 95% of the sample at an average age of 20 for our ten-year follow-up, with a 15-year follow-up now in progress. Once the latter is completed, we will have thorough information through the age span of the mid-20s.

As an example of the importance of considering female-specific manifestations of development — and as a sobering reminder of the devastating impairments that can accrue from a history of ADHD — I emphasize key findings.[19] At our adolescent follow-up we found evidence for significant and often large impairments in the ADHD sample within each of the 11 domains we assessed, spanning academics, peer relationships, comorbidities, global impairment, self-perceptions, and family functioning.[20] Math performance remained strikingly low, as did performance on tests of executive functioning.[21] In addition, only a depressingly small number of the ADHD sample was, at this time, showing positive/resilient functioning in adolescence.[22] In short, by the teen years ADHD-related impairments were, if anything, stronger than they were in childhood, even though for many participants some of the initial ADHD symptoms were being shed.

Five years later, by early adulthood, similar impairments persisted. In addition, we found that executive functions, measured during childhood, were especially important predictors of functional impairment.[23, 24] Furthermore, and crucially, we assessed additional domains of functioning linked to the young-adult developmental level of the participants, including the area of self-harm.[25, 26] (Note that it is essential in longitudinal research to (a) use parallel measures to those from earlier data waves, whenever possible, to reveal patterns of change over time without confounding old scales with new scales, but at the same time to (b) add developmentally relevant measures to supplement those utilized previously.)

Here, findings were particularly devastating. In general, we had found that girls initially diagnosed with the Inattentive form of ADHD were as likely to show impairment, later on, as those with the Combined form. Yet for the group of girls who had displayed not only inattention but high levels of impulsivity during childhood (i.e., the Combined type), their risk for serious suicide attempts was nearly 23% by young adulthood (far higher than for the purely Inattentive and comparison groups), and their rates of moderate to severe non-suicidal self-injurious behavior were over 50% — again, much higher than for the other subgroups. In short, girls with ADHD were at risk for high levels of self-destructive actions across the life span, far more than boys.[27] The lasting legacy of early problems with impulsivity, particularly during the already-difficult transition to adolescence experienced by girls in general,[28] portends a pattern of internalizing behavior and self-harm in girls with ADHD at levels far beyond those experienced by boys. Moreover, aggressive behavior and poor response inhibition during adolescence explained the risk for non-suicidal self-injury in our sample, whereas anxiety and depression during adolescence were mediators of the long-term risk for suicide attempts.[29] In addition, rates of early trauma — including physical abuse, sexual abuse, and neglect — were particularly predictive of the sample's risk for suicidal behavior.[30]

There are several morals to this story. First, when ADHD exists in girls, the long-term consequences are devastating and in key respects different from those of boys. For girls, impulsivity and its consequences predict levels of self-destruction not seen in male samples, bespeaking the urgent need for debunking the still-persistent myths that ADHD does not really exist in females or is not of much real importance in girls and women. Second, clinicians and research investigators alike must pay careful attention to the growing numbers of girls and women with ADHD, demanding careful evaluations to avoid potential problems of rampant over diagnosis[31] and emphasizing gender-specific manifestations, pathways, and impairments. Third, accessible, sensitive, and clinically relevant information on girls and women with ADHD must be available to readers from all walks of life.

It is here where the new edition of "Understanding Girls with ADHD" comes to the fore. In this expanded and updated book, Kathleen Nadeau, Ellen Littman, and Patricia Quinn rise to the occasion and deliver a comprehensive, up-to-date, and readable book that illuminates the complexity of ADHD in girls and women, both across the lifespan and across multiple domains of life (e.g., home, school, the workplace, close relationships).

Blending clinical examples, case material, and a masterful synthesis of research findings around the world, the authors reveal the roots of ADHD in females during the preschool years, also summarizing relevant causal factors, and display the highly individualized journeys through childhood, adolescence, and adulthood that these girls and women face. The book's latter chapters make use of the information on ADHD and development and provide a synthesis of the kinds of treatment strategies needed to intervene with the complex issues faced by girls and families who struggle with ADHD. The authors' working through the executive functioning deficits experienced by so many girls with ADHD — and their deployment of vivid examples of right vs. wrong ways of approaching such problems — will be of great importance for large numbers of families. Even more, the authors emphasize that ADHD rarely exists in a vacuum and that understanding and treating comorbid disorders is essential.

"Understanding Girls with ADHD" does not shy away from key areas of controversy. How, for example, can a family know whether it's ADHD or another set of problems that's the primary issue? How does one deal with the potential use of medication, which is plagued by bad press and abundant myths but which can, as part of a multi-faceted treatment plan, provide great benefit if the right dose is found and if the doctor works with the family to monitor positive effects and side effects carefully? What about long-term risk for eating pathology, substance abuse, and other difficult areas of impairment of salience for girls? How can girls and their families break through the thicket of negative expectations and sometimes-toxic family interactions to pave the way for a different set of outcomes?

Clearly, ADHD does not look the same across different individuals, especially girls. "Understanding Girls with ADHD" emphasizes the multiple ways in which ADHD can manifest itself across different people, families, and ages. Always sensitive, and without hesitation in providing an authoritative tone, this book will empower girls and their families in ways that are sorely needed. Its emphasis on gender-specific manifestations of ADHD and its inclusion of practical means of attacking the executive-function deficits that plague girls and women with ADHD will ensure its continued status as a core guidebook.

Written with compassion and sensitivity, and full of the clinical wisdom that accompanies years of experience on the front lines, "Understanding Girls with ADHD" is the go-to book for those needing guidance, support, and knowledge about female manifestations of ADHD. Given my own work related to developmental psychopathology in general[32] and ADHD in particular — including recognition of the still-prevalent stigma that clings to many forms of mental disorder[33] — I welcome this edition as a means of providing clarity, enlightenment, and guidance to the millions of girls and their families who can and will benefit from its sage words. ADHD is too often the source of real impairment rather than an inevitable hidden gift. Still, as the book makes abundantly clear, there is no need to perpetuate blame, shame, and stigma. Instead, empowerment, knowledge, support, and evidence-based treatments are what every family needs.

— Stephen P. Hinshaw, Ph.D.,
University of California, Berkeley, 2014

Understanding Girls with ADHD

How they feel and why they do what they do

CHAPTER ONE

We've Come a Long Way, But There's Still Far to Go

A FEW SHORT DECADES AGO, there was no such thing as a girl with Attention Deficit Hyperactivity Disorder (ADHD). Although it existed in girls, it went unrecognized and was called by many other names. A girl may have been labeled a "tomboy" with skinned knees, and everyone hoped she'd settle down and outgrow it. Or maybe she was a sweet, shy daydreamer. "We're not worried," her parent might have said, "she'll find a good husband to take care of her." Maybe she was seen as a social butterfly, always getting in trouble for talking in class. "She's a smart girl, she's just not applying herself," a teacher would remark. Perhaps she was fiery and argumentative, rejecting her mother's admonitions to be more ladylike.

Parents and teachers had their excuses and opinions, but what was it like for the girls with ADHD. How did they feel?

WHAT IS ADHD LIKE FOR GIRLS?

The following poignant lament eloquently expresses the experience of one of the countless girls with ADHD who grew up before ADHD was recognized in girls. "I Wish My Mother Had Known" was written in the mid-1990s by a recently diagnosed middle-aged woman — one of the sweet, shy daydreamers. At the time this poem was written, women with ADHD were taking the initiative to seek diagnosis, while most girls still languished in the classroom, overlooked and misunderstood, suffering silently.

I WISH MY MOTHER HAD KNOWN

By Mary H.

I wish my mother had known
that I was actually very smart.
I wish my mother had known
that I needed more attention.

I wish my mother had known
that I went to school every day as a little girl,
in fear and dread
at the prospect of being shamed
and humiliated in class.

I wish my mother had known
that my low self-esteem and
lack of physical affection at home
would lead to rampant promiscuity.

I wish my mother had known
that someday I would have to
compete in the world,
and that being married
was not going to make me safe.

I wish my mother had known how desperately
I needed stimulation and attainable challenges.
(Expectations for me were very low,
so even I was surprised when I realized
that I love a challenge!)

I wish my mother had known
that I was too sensitive and shy and embarrassed
to have my needs met.

I wish my mother had known
that I could not easily either fall asleep or wake up,
and that I had no control over that.

I wish my mother had known
that being put into the dumb classes,
in spite of my consistently high IQ tests,
was humiliating,
and caused me to not even bother to try.

I wish my mother had known
that having only one friend
was not normal and
might have signaled other problems.

I wish my mother had known
that leaving the house unzipped, buttoned wrong,
or without my lunch or books, was a signal.

I wish my mother had known
that I had a huge curiosity about life,
but that I could not absorb it
in the context of public school.

I wish my mother had known
that my artistic and creative skills
were important,
and could have sustained me
had I been encouraged to develop them.

I wish my mother had known
that I could not organize my room.

I wish my mother had known
what we know now.
She didn't. She did her best,
and I hope that she knows
how very much I love her.

Mary's poem can almost serve as an outline for this book. She details the behaviors that should have signaled to her parents and teachers that there were underlying problems:

- School phobia or avoidance
- Low self-esteem
- Low academic performance, despite high IQ and creativity
- Poor organizational skills, messiness
- Sleep problems
- Shyness
- Poor social skills
- Disheveled appearance, grooming problems
- Withdrawal in the classroom

Mary describes the unwitting assumptions that allowed both her parents and teachers to overlook and undervalue her talents and abilities; and she relates not only the causes, but suggests possible solutions that could have helped her to overcome her limitations:

- Recognition and understanding of her struggles
- Positive attention and affection to offset daily assaults on her self-esteem
- Affirmation and encouragement
- Acknowledgement of her strengths
- An ADHD-friendly learning environment
- Appropriate stimulation and challenges
- Assistance with structure and organization
- Help with chronic sleep problems
- Support to develop more assertiveness
- Recognition of and support for social challenges

OUR WORK IS NOT YET DONE

Though the identification of girls with ADHD has progressed markedly, our work is not yet done. A recent study found that teachers continue to identify many more males than females, most likely because males are more disruptive in the classroom.[1] However, even more troubling are the results of another study that found that teachers and parents were more likely to refer boys rather than girls with ADHD for services, even when they reportedly exhibited identical behaviors.[2]

Why is it that teachers can easily recognize boys with ADHD, but seem to overlook the differences between girls with ADHD and others? Perhaps it is because they have greater difficulty understanding that the feelings and behaviors typically seen in these girls are actually signs of ADHD. These signs include patterns such as hyper-talkativeness, blurting out answers without raising one's hand, social withdrawal, a tendency to miss or misunderstand directions, arriving at school without necessary materials, messiness, disorganization, test anxiety, late or missing assignments, and forgetfulness. Even an intense, anxious hyper-focus on schoolwork may signal a girl with ADHD who is frantically attempting to compensate for her difficulties. Teachers are less likely to refer girls who forget their lunch money, lose their homework, or seem unmotivated in class, perhaps because the only ones to suffer from these behaviors are the girls themselves, but also because teachers are not aware that these patterns are typical of girls with ADHD.

Mothers seem to be much more aware than teachers of the differences in their ADHD daughters' behaviors when compared to other girls.[3] This finding highlights a major obstacle to diagnosing girls, since ADHD symptoms must negatively impact functioning and be reported in more than one setting. A mother may be very aware of her daughter's ADHD, but if the teacher doesn't recognize it, the diagnosis may not be made. And worse, the mother may be blamed for her reports of problems at home since these behaviors are not being observed at school.

The authors' clinical experience is that girls try much harder to conform to their teachers' expectations, masking their ADHD struggles until later when even their greatest efforts cannot overcome their ADHD challenges. Changes in the DSM-5, published in 2013,[4] however, should contribute to improved identification of these girls with ADHD. New DSM-5 guidelines allow for a diagnosis of ADHD if symptoms emerge as late as age 12. (Previously, the cut-off was age seven.) This change will have a significant impact upon the diagnosis of girls because there is evidence that girls' ADHD symptoms often emerge later.[5]

USE OF SELF-REPORT SCALES

In contrast to studies that only use scales completed by parents and teachers and as a result recognize ADHD in more boys than girls, studies that use self-report scales as part of the diagnostic process for ADHD uncover nearly equal numbers of males and females.[6] Self-report on the part of girls is critical, because for most girls ADHD is an internalized disorder, that is, a disorder that impacts the individual in ways that may not be easily observed by others.

The authors of this book have developed and recently revised a Girls ADHD Self-Report Scale to allow girls the opportunity to describe their own experience as a girl with ADHD. This scale can be found in the Appendix at the back of this book.

There are not yet standardized norms for this self-report scale; therefore, it should not be used as a diagnostic tool. However, it can be very useful as a means of opening up a more detailed and comprehensive discussion with girls about how they are impacted by ADHD.

OUR EVOLVING UNDERSTANDING OF ADHD

Now that we are doing a much better job of identifying girls with ADHD, our primary focus turns to efforts to better understand girls, how they feel, why they do what they do, and how we can help them feel and function better. There is still so much that we don't know. How are girls with ADHD similar to boys with the disorder? How do they differ? Do they need different supports and treatment approaches? What is the outcome of ADHD in girls over time?

In the past fifteen years, there have been important developments in our still evolving understanding of ADHD. These developments are not specifically related to girls, but are highly relevant because these new ways of conceptualizing ADHD apply to girls as well as boys. Below, we briefly introduce these new conceptualizations of ADHD.

ADHD is now considered to be a developmental disorder

Our more recent view of ADHD places emphasis upon impaired cognitive functions rather than upon hyperactivity, impulsivity and distractibility. To reflect this new understanding, the DSM-5 classifies ADHD as a "developmental disorder" rather than as a "behavior disorder of childhood" as it was classified earlier.[7] Our focus has turned toward the impact of ADHD upon cognitive functions and away from our earlier emphasis upon hyperactivity, impulsivity and disruptive behaviors. This shift will naturally lead to easier identification of girls who are less likely to be hyperactive, impulsive and disruptive.

ADHD – A focus on executive functions

Dr. Thomas Brown of Yale University was a very early leader in the shift to a focus on executive functions as the core issues of ADHD. In his research on highly intelligent students with ADHD, he found that while some of them were hyperactive and impulsive, all of them shared core executive function issues as well as issues related to mood. He developed the Brown ADD Scales,[8] questionnaires that assess an individual's difficulties in areas such as getting started on a task, sustaining effort on a challenging task, becoming distracted from a task, regulating emotions (low frustration tolerance, emotional overreactions, mood and anxiety issues), and memory difficulties.

A great deal more has been written in recent years about the executive functions of the brain as core components of ADHD — executive functions such as ability to organize, to plan, to self-monitor, to maintain time awareness, to problem-solve and shift focus intentionally. All of these executive function issues greatly impact girls with ADHD and will be explored in later chapters of this book.

ADHD as a "foundational disorder" related to other disorders

ADHD is a complex condition that is associated with many other disorders. Dr. Thomas Brown, mentioned above for his work on executive function issues, has called ADHD a "foundational disorder" because childhood ADHD seems to provide a foundation that sets the stage for the development of many other psychiatric disorders as children grow and mature. Studies have demonstrated that adults with ADHD have a 70% probability of having one or more coexisting psychiatric conditions.[9]

We have long known that anxiety and mood disorders are frequent among girls with ADHD and that ADHD often precedes the development of bipolar disorder. ADHD is commonly found in combination with various learning disorders, with written language disorder nearly always present when ADHD and reading disorders are found together. ADHD brings with it a risk of substance abuse disorders, borderline personality disorder and mood dysregulation disorders. In the years since the publication of our first edition of *Understanding Girls with ADHD*, there has been a growing, now widespread recognition that girls with ADHD are at risk of eating disorders, especially binge eating disorder. These coexisting issues will be discussed in greater detail in the chapters that follow.

UNDERSTANDING GIRLS WITH ADHD

Above, we have outlined changes in our thinking about ADHD that applies to both males and females. Now, let's turn our attention to developments specific to girls.

Disabilities exist within and are influenced by social and biological contexts. Girls are biologically different; they socialize and verbalize differently; and they live in a society that, even today, has different expectations for males and females. ADHD in girls needs to be viewed through the lens of these biological and social gender differences.

Gender and diagnostic criteria for ADHD

Despite the gains that have been made in the diagnosis of ADHD in girls, challenges still persist. The long-standing, male-based, diagnostic criteria are very slow to change. One recent study[10] reported that mothers of children with ADHD view the standard diagnostic criteria as more descriptive of boys than girls with ADHD. Consequently, even current research may be limited in its ability to contribute to a greater understanding of ADHD in females if it continues to use these male-based criteria.

Gender and behavioral manifestations of ADHD

Most studies seem to be in agreement that girls with ADHD show significantly fewer conduct problems or oppositional defiant disorders than do boys with ADHD.[11, 12] However, there is a downside to these findings. Since, as discussed earlier, this decreased incidence of behavior problems seems to lead to a lower rate of teacher referral, penalizing girls who may have significant problems with inattention and distractibility, but who do not draw attention to themselves.[13]

Likewise, there is general agreement across studies that girls with ADHD are less hyperactive than are boys.[14] One question that has yet to be raised is whether hyperactivity is the same in boys and girls. For example, clinical observation suggests that hyperactivity in girls may be manifested more through hyperverbalization and emotional excitability/reactivity, which are more difficult to measure and quantify than motoric hyperactivity. Thus, girls may show fewer or different symptoms, but be just as impaired.

Gender and social challenges of ADHD

While social challenges are commonplace in children with ADHD, girls appear to face even more social challenges than their male counterparts.[15] Girls with ADHD tend to alienate their peers.[16] Studies demonstrate that girls with ADHD experience more peer rejection than do boys with ADHD[17] and that as they get older they are less popular with their peers.[18]

Unlike the physical aggression more common among boys, girls tend to engage in verbal aggression, gossip and social exclusion.[19] Girls with ADHD are also often the target of this relational aggression. Girls with combined type ADHD are more likely to be socially rejected by their non-ADHD girls, while girls with inattentive type ADHD are more likely to be "socially neglected," i.e., ignored or left out rather than being the target of active rejection.[20]

Gender and greater self-blame, lower self-esteem

Girls with ADHD tend to internalize criticism they receive from peers, teachers and parents, leading to a strong sense of shame and self-blame. Research suggests that women, after they have progressed beyond their impulse-driven adolescent years, are much more likely than men to feel a sense of shame or humiliation as they look back on their earlier impulsive behaviors,[21] a finding supported by another study that suggests that women with ADHD struggle much more with a negative self-image than do men,[22] despite no reported differences in impairment between the men and women. Strong cultural factors are surely impacting the low self-esteem reported more often by females than males.[23]

Gender and hormonal influences on ADHD

Hormonal changes occurring at puberty affect emotional volatility, leading many girls with ADHD to become emotionally hyper-reactive. Huessy writes that behavioral problems for many girls with ADHD only begin after puberty, accompanied by an increase in emotional over-reactivity, mood swings, and impulsivity.[24] This is a critical finding because many of these girls do not meet the DSM-5 requirement that evidence of ADHD problems must exist prior to 12 years of age in order to receive an ADHD diagnosis.

Gender and ADHD after puberty

The rates of anxiety and depression in ADHD girls increase as they pass through late adolescence into young adulthood. Girls with ADHD were found to be 5.4 times more likely to be diagnosed with major depression than girls without the condition.[25] In addition, adolescent girls with ADHD were found to be doing less well in general when compared to girls without ADHD. The majority of adolescent girls with ADHD were found to be poorly adjusted, with continued ADHD symptoms, behavior problems, internalizing problems (i.e., depressive and anxiety symptoms), and problems with social skills, peer relationships, and academic functioning. Only 16% of girls with ADHD were found to have overall positive adjustment in adolescence in contrast to the 86% of non-ADHD girls with an overall positive adjustment.[26]

Gender and long-term risks associated with ADHD

Because girls with ADHD are less physically aggressive, less disruptive, less hyperactive and less defiant, girls with ADHD were viewed for many years as having a paler, less serious version of ADHD. In the past decade, however, studies have demonstrated, to the contrary, that girls with ADHD demonstrate a far higher risk than boys of developing serious psychiatric disorders as they mature. A study by Rucklidge and Tannock suggests that adolescent females with ADHD have more psychological distress than their male counterparts. When compared to males, girls with ADHD report more anxiety, more distress, more depressive symptoms, and were more likely to hold a belief that they had little control over the events in their lives. They were also at risk for more psychological impairments.[27] In a study of children with ADHD that were reassessed in adulthood, girls were more than twice as likely as boys with ADHD to have a psychiatric admission in adulthood and were more likely to have a lifetime diagnosis of a mood disorder, substance use disorder or schizophrenia.[28] In addition, a recent study reported that girls with ADHD are at a much greater risk of making a suicide attempt compared to girls without ADHD.[29]

THE GOOD NEWS

Parents of girls with ADHD may understandably react with alarm to the likelihood that these other serious mental health conditions may develop later. What is important for parents to understand is that the emergence and severity of these various coexisting conditions can be reduced by early identification of ADHD followed by interventions. Successful interventions include increased structure and support at home and in a girl's school environment, parent training to learn positive, effective parenting approaches, development of brain-healthy daily habits including exercise, sleep, nutrition, stress reduction, social and environmental interventions, and medication.

A FEW WORDS FOR WORRIED PARENTS

Parents can have a powerful positive effect on their daughters with ADHD. It's important to keep in mind that while certain characteristics of ADHD can prove problematic for girls with ADHD and their families, many of these same tendencies have an adaptive side as well. Parents can acknowledge the challenges of ADHD, but can also help their daughters reframe their difficulties as opportunities. Girls that are non-linear thinkers, who do not feel constrained by social conventions, can find unusual ways of solving problems and creative ways of re-thinking things. Girls that are daydreamers may discover that their rich imagination becomes the fuel for creative writing. Those with high energy will be tireless in pursuing a project of interest; they can be the most dedicated and determined volunteers for a cause they believe in. Their symptoms can be reframed so that they don't just focus on their challenges but appreciate themselves as unique and endowed with valuable strengths as well.

Parents need to teach their daughters that although they may find school a poor fit for their strengths and interests, a much broader range of choices awaits them after school years are through. We need to help girls with ADHD understand that the path to success and satisfaction lies in understanding themselves and in seeking or creating an environment that is a good match for their unique selves.

It's important for parents to understand that girls with ADHD who believe they can succeed academically are more likely to have positive outcomes. Girls who feel confident about their academic competence, regardless of their actual achievement, experience increased academic success over time. These girls will have fewer problems with mood, anxiety, or behavior problems, as well as a reduced risk of substance abuse.[30] A belief in their abilities should be consistently and enthusiastically fostered by parents and teachers; the potential outcome is that these girls are more likely to remain invested in school. These findings suggest that one of the most powerful interventions that parents can offer is a consistent sense of hope.

It's also important for parents to understand that girls who have been parented with consistent discipline and appropriate limits have a greater likelihood of positive outcomes.[31] When their experiences are validated by their families; they are more likely to develop a strong sense of self-respect. A supportive and attuned family can teach the skills necessary for girls with ADHD to communicate their needs assertively and advocate for themselves.

While it's all too easy to catch your daughter misbehaving and disappointing you, it's important to make the effort to catch her being good as often as possible. Being "good" doesn't have to mean being tidy or making good grades; it can mean a wonderful smile, a helpful gesture, a friendly remark, or a determined effort, even if success is not reached. Noticing and complimenting the behaviors that you value will be the reinforcement she needs to perform the same behavior again. Genuine praise for a sincere effort is a wonderful boost to self-esteem. Your daughter needs to know that, rather than being silenced by her shame, that you want to empower her to be heard — and that you're listening.

CONCLUSION

Our goals in this book are to alert parents, teachers, and the professional community about the more subtle signs of ADHD in girls, to highlight the risks associated with ADHD in girls, to explore more gender-specific ways to treat girls with ADHD, and to focus on the needs of these girls in all aspects of their lives.

After reading this book, we want parents, educators, and other professionals to understand that:

1. ADHD is a complex disorder and that it is almost always accompanied by other disorders that must be treated in conjunction with ADHD.

2. Parents can provide protection against, or reduce the impact of, many of these conditions through appropriate treatment, parent support, educational accommodations, and the creation of ADHD-friendly environments at home, at school, and in their daughter's social environments.

3. Raising a daughter with ADHD is a challenging but potentially very rewarding enterprise. Parents should get the best help, and seek it early in their daughter's life, in order to learn positive, effective, parenting strategies.

In the chapters that follow, we will guide the reader to a fuller understanding of what is going on in girls with ADHD – biologically, socially, emotionally, and academically. We will discuss how girls are impacted by ADHD at various developmental stages, but more importantly, we will provide practical information about how parents, educators, and other professionals can help these girls function well in their daily lives and develop an appreciation of their strengths while learning how to problem-solve to meet the challenges posed by ADHD. We have a long way to go, so let's get started.

CHAPTER TWO

Learning More About the Brain and Other Biological Factors Influencing ADHD

IN THIS CHAPTER, WE WILL take you on a brief tour of the brain to understand the basics about how it develops, how it typically functions, and how it is affected by ADHD. The key message for parents reading this chapter is that ADHD is a real, brain-based disorder, not a disorder invented as an excuse for poor parenting, misbehavior, or academic struggles. Just as important, we don't want parents to feel that because ADHD is brain-based that there is nothing to be done aside from taking medication. We mold and develop our brains through the activities that we engage in. Our brains function better or worse based upon the brain-healthy daily habits we engage in as well as the environment in which we are functioning. In this chapter, we describe brain differences that are associated with ADHD symptoms. In later chapters, we will introduce multiple ways in which we can influence and improve brain functioning.

The brain is an amazingly complex organ. While we are beginning to understand some of the brain's power and functions, much more remains a mystery. What we do know is that ADHD is a brain-based disorder. Research has documented differences in brain structure, brain chemistry, and brain wave patterns in those with ADHD.

NEW TECHNOLOGIES OPEN A WINDOW TO THE BRAIN

We now have technologies to look inside the brain in a noninvasive fashion, allowing us to learn about the brain's structure and function. PET scans can measure the level of activity in particular regions of the brain. CAT scans can determine the size and structure of different parts of the brain, while fMRIs can tell us exactly which parts of the brain are activated or turned off as we perform various mental tasks. EEGs can track brain wave patterns in different regions of the brain. In part, due to these technologies, our understanding of ADHD continues to increase and evolve.

Formerly, we classified ADHD as a behavior disorder of childhood in response to the most noticeable behaviors — hyperactivity, impulsivity, and distractibility. We now know that such patterns are true of only some children with ADHD. Your daughter with ADHD may or may not exhibit hyperactivity and impulsivity, but there are other ADHD-related problems that she will encounter including problems with self-regulation[1] and executive functioning.[2] We now classify ADHD as a developmental disorder (DSM-5) rather than a behavioral disorder. Developmental disorders are those that affect behavioral and cognitive functioning, whose beginnings occur before birth, and continue during early childhood development.[3]

BRAIN DEVELOPMENT

In order to better understand ADHD in girls, it's important to first understand about the brain and its formation and development, taking note of differences that have been seen in areas that control attention, planning, working memory, emotions, and motivation.

In the typically developing brain, billions of brain cells (neurons) arise from a single layer of cells — the outer cell layer of the embryo (the ectoderm) — during the third and fourth weeks after conception, a time when most women don't even know that they are pregnant. During the early weeks of pregnancy, these cells rapidly multiply. Remarkably, somewhere around the sixth month of pregnancy, the brain already contains the same number of cells as the adult brain. Beyond the sixth month, brain cells continue to multiply, and by the time of birth a baby has many more brain cells than it will have as an adult. These brain cells will gradually decrease in number with unneeded cells dying off as the brain develops specialized areas of function.

Meanwhile, a rich network of fibers develops to connect these specialized brain areas enabling them to act in concert to perform complex functions. This rich network is necessary to transmit brain signals to carry on the work of the brain.

One of the most important networks of connective fibers (the corpus callosum) facilitates communication and coordination between the two hemispheres of the brain. Neural networks efficiently send signals from one area of the brain to another, a bit like super-highways connecting smaller roads in individual neighborhoods of the brain. While most areas of the brain stop growing and begin the process of cell pruning and specialization, one important area at the base of the brain, the cerebellum, continues to develop until a baby is 10 or 11 months old. The prefrontal cortex (PFC), located behind the forehead, is the seat of higher-level cognitive functions such as planning, decision-making, self-monitoring, and self-control. This is the last area to complete its development, sometime during late adolescence.[4] We'll return to a further discussion of the PFC later in this chapter as it is an area of the brain significantly implicated in symptoms of ADHD.

THE DEVELOPING BRAIN AND ADHD RISK FACTORS

As you might imagine, during the prenatal period, as the brain undergoes rapid development, it is particularly vulnerable to damage. Prenatal brain insults can result from numerous factors including bleeding during the first trimester of pregnancy, maternal stress, maternal smoking, alcohol or cocaine abuse, and complications during delivery.[5, 6] Following birth, a rapid and vulnerable period of brain growth continues to approximately four years of age. During this period of development, the brain is most susceptible to injury due to nutritional deficiencies, trauma, infection, and environmental toxins such as lead and pesticides.[7] Prematurity and low birth weight are further complicating factors that lead to later problems with almost half of these infants experiencing learning disabilities and ADHD.[8] Genes also affect developing brain structure and functioning.

ADHD has been shown to be genetic and highly hereditary.[9] If one or both parents have ADHD, there's a high likelihood that their child will have it as well.[10]

EVIDENCE FOR A NEUROBIOLOGICAL BASIS FOR ADHD

The newer technologies that allow us to view inside the brain have helped us to better understand the PFC and the function of different areas of the PFC that are involved in ADHD. One part of the PFC seems to regulate attention, planning and working memory; another part is involved in cognitive control, and a third part of the PFC is used to regulate our emotions and motivation.[11]

Slower development in nearly all brain regions and structural abnormalities within the PFC, specifically, has been seen in children and adolescents with ADHD.[12] In those children and adolescents with ADHD, the cortex in areas that contain networks that modulate attention and executive functioning was found to be thinner when compared to children without ADHD. Children whose ADHD had a worse outcome as they matured were seen to have *fixed* thinning resulting in a continued compromise of attentional networks, while this same area (the right parietal cortex) was seen to ultimately develop a normal thickness in children with ADHD who had a better outcome as they aged.[13] In a study of slightly older children (10 to 18 years) with ADHD,[14] the typical developmental pattern of overproduction of brain cells before puberty and pruning during adolescence, as measured by cortical thickness, was found to be similar to a control group although maturation occurred much later in the ADHD group. Long-term follow-up studies suggest that all children with ADHD have delayed cortical maturation. And that only some of these children with better outcomes eventually show complete cortical maturation in adolescence or later.[15] In fact, continuing ADHD symptoms in adults can be predicted by the presence of continued cortical thinning during adolescence in regions of the brain believed to modulate attention and executive functioning.[16]

What can we conclude from these studies? First, that the differences found in the size of various brain structures suggest that ADHD is, in the majority of cases, a lifelong condition linked to developments in the prenatal period and during infancy when development of these brain structures is taking place. Second, that these alterations in brain structures are the direct result of influences on the brain during early development. While the origin of these changes are unknown, they are most likely the result of genetic predisposition or insults to the brain from other sources such as prematurity, infections, or exposure to lead. Third, it is also important to note that, while many of these studies found smaller size in various structures, none of the studies found any evidence of brain damage. Lastly, it should be pointed out that bad parenting, poor schools, lazy teachers, etc., occurring at a later period in the child's life, could not have caused these differences in brain structures.

DIFFERENCES IN BRAIN STRUCTURE AND CONNECTIVITY WHEN ADHD IS PRESENT

Numerous studies have documented structural differences in ADHD brains in specific areas including the PFC,[17,18] the cerebellum, and the corpus callosum (the bridge between the two sides of the brain).[19,20] Despite this growing evidence, it is troubling that healthcare professionals and members of the press, as well as those in the general population, continue to profess the opinion that ADHD is not a real disorder, but rather the result of bad parenting, lazy teachers, poor schools, or a fast-paced society.

The findings of impaired PFC network functioning are extremely important because the functions of the PFC are typically impaired in those with ADHD. Impaired neural networks connecting the PFC to other key areas of the brain arise during brain development and contribute to the life-long symptoms of ADHD.[21]

CHEMICAL NEUROTRANSMITTERS

Differences in ADHD brains are not only related to brain structure but also to brain chemistry. Chemicals called neurotransmitters are secreted by brain cells (neurons); these chemicals cross the synapse, a tiny gap between brain cells, carrying a message to the adjacent cell. A single neuron may have as many as 1,000 to 10,000 points of contact with other cells. Each neuron in the brain can receive these chemical messengers from many other neurons. While no single area of the brain can account for all the symptoms of ADHD, the neuronal pathways that rely on dopamine and norepinephrine have been associated with the behaviors we see in those with ADHD.

Studies of the brains of boys with and without ADHD found that boys with ADHD had slightly smaller brains with decreased volume in exactly those areas of the brain heavily depending upon the neurochemical dopamine,[22, 23] providing valuable information about which chemical neurotransmitters may be involved in ADHD. Shifts in levels of dopamine and norepinephrine may lead to fluctuations in brain function, particularly the PFC.[24] Many of the medications effective in reducing ADHD symptoms increase the amount of dopamine and norepinephrine in the PFC and other areas of the brain.

DIFFERENCES IN THE BRAIN ARE PRESENT AS EARLY AS PRESCHOOL YEARS

Although research looking at the brains of young children is sparse, it's important to take note of those differences that have been found. Studies providing insights into brain differences associated with ADHD have almost exclusively focused on children ages seven and older. However, in 2011, a study of preschoolers looked at regions of the brain important for both cognitive and motor control and found that these brain regions were smaller in children with ADHD than in typically developing children. Researchers examined brain images in preschoolers (ages four and five) both with and without symptoms of ADHD, specifically looking at those areas of the brain known to correlate with hyperactivity and impulsivity. They found that these brain areas in children with ADHD were significantly reduced in size compared to the children without ADHD symptoms.[25] One of the most important implications of this research is that it provides more evidence that ADHD differences exist very early in a child's development and that ADHD symptoms are not caused by later social or environmental factors.

GENDER DIFFERENCES IN BRAIN STRUCTURE

While most of the brain research at this point has involved only boys with ADHD, nevertheless, it remains valuable in understanding what is going on in the brain of a person with ADHD.

This research clearly shows an involvement of the frontal and prefrontal cortex of the brain as well as the areas to which they connect in the deeper parts of the brain (subcortical/striatum areas). These are the areas specifically linked to motivation and emotional control — two brain functions that are adversely affected when a person has ADHD.[26] The executive functions of the brain — attention, impulse control, goal-orientation, and problem-solving — are also known to be dependent on the prefrontal lobes and these subcortical connections.[27]

But what are the gender differences, if any, seen in the female versus the male brain? To answer this question, let's look at several other studies. One such study measured the size of various brain structures in 30 children (15 males and 15 females) ages seven to 11 years. This study found that the brain at this age is 95% the volume of an adult brain. As in other areas of the body, the female brain as a whole was usually slightly smaller than the male brain, but the size was proportional and not significantly different.[28] The female brain usually weighs less than the male brain for the same reason that her liver and kidneys are smaller and weigh less. Her head size is smaller, just as her foot size is smaller.

This proportionally smaller size relationship held up in most areas in the brain, but there were some significant exceptions. Certain areas of the female brain were larger than in the male brain, including the caudate, hippocampus, and palladium. The size of these structures has been noted to be inversely proportional to the degree of hyperactivity (e.g. the smaller the caudate the more hyperactivity seen), and is, therefore, probably the reason that girls (with larger caudate nuclei) are generally less hyperactive than boys. Conversely, the amygdala was noted to be disproportionately smaller in the female brain. Emotional disorders such as anxiety and depression are linked to activity in the amygdala. Differences in these structures of the limbic system (seat of emotional regulation) would be expected to be one of the reasons for the differing patterns of coexisting conditions seen in females versus males, and might also be the underpinning of the variable symptom presentations in certain disorders, including ADHD.

DIFFERENCES IN BRAIN DEVELOPMENT BETWEEN GIRLS AND BOYS WITH ADHD

In this same study, other differences were also found between the brains of girls and boys with ADHD. Because the PFC is implicated in so many of the challenges related to ADHD, it is important to note that the PFC in girls with ADHD appeared to have reached adult volume, suggesting that girls had more clearly defined areas of function earlier than the PFC of boys, in which cell pruning had not yet taken place. (You'll recall we mentioned early in this chapter that cell pruning, the dying off of unused cells, takes place as the brain matures and develops more defined areas of specific functioning.) Thus with earlier maturation, executive functioning skills would be seen earlier in females than males, but skills (and deficits) would be more fixed with fewer improvements seen in these areas in girls over time.

These findings confirm earlier studies that demonstrated that the brains of boys have a greater overproduction of cells and decrease in size as a result of pruning during adolescence. It is this pruning that seems to assure an increase in specificity, the more efficient functioning of neuron pathways in the brain, and a decrease in symptoms. Therefore, it seems that the earlier maturation of these areas in the brains of girls results in more fixed deficits than in boys' brains, where overproduction of cells and later pruning, allow boys to receive a greater opportunity for functional improvement and symptom reduction in later adolescence. The bottom line is that girls' brains mature earlier, but have less opportunity to overcome impairments later. Thus their fixed levels of deficits related to the specialization of the PFC and related brain areas occurs earlier than in boys.

GENDER DIFFERENCES IN DOPAMINE RECEPTORS

ADHD is currently thought to be the result of impairments in the dopamine and norepinephrine neurotransmitter pathways in the brain. Specific receptors control transmission in these areas of the brain, thus modulating behaviors, and have been shown to be affected by gender. Animal studies give us clues as to what happens during brain development in female versus male brains. One such study assessed the number of dopamine receptors in male and female rats from puberty into adulthood. It found that males had greater overproduction and elimination of these receptors than did females.[29] These gender differences in the development of the dopamine system may have significant implications regarding the gender differences seen in ADHD.

As research has suggested, the overproduction of dopamine receptors during prepubertal development may help explain why males have more hyperactive symptoms and other disorders such as Tourette syndrome. Likewise, the extensive pruning that occurs during adolescence might help explain why symptoms of hyperactivity diminish in males after puberty. And most importantly, the fact that density does not recede in females may explain why ADHD symptoms are more likely to persist in females after puberty. It is the pruning as a result of overproduction that allows for the ability of the brain to set up more effective systems that correct previous deficits and improve functioning.

For girls, the lack of overproduction and pruning deprives their brains of this opportunity and results in more fixed deficits and persistent symptoms. There is also emerging evidence that abnormal regulation of these patterns of brain development, as a result of sex hormone differences, can be associated with differences in psychological and behavioral disorders in males and females. This research will be discussed further in the section on ADHD in puberty.

EFFECTS OF ESTROGEN ON BRAIN DEVELOPMENT

While the effect of estrogen on the sex organs has been known for years, it has only recently been discovered that estrogen also affects the brain. Both boy and girl fetuses are subjected to high levels of estrogen while in the uterus during the early phases of brain development. After birth, both males and females produce estrogen. However, females have as much as three to ten times the levels of estrogen as males until the years leading up to menopause. It is in girls, especially, that we must consider the effects of higher levels of estrogen on brain maturation and function. McEwen and coworkers reported in 1997 that ovarian steroids have effects throughout the brain, including on the dopamine and serotonin levels.[30] Estrogen has also been shown to stimulate a significant increase in dopamine and serotonin receptors.[31]

SENSITIVITY TO CHANGES IN ESTROGEN LEVELS

Receptors and binding sites are important because the more receptors we have, the more responsive our system will be to even a small amount of a neurotransmitter. In conditions such as ADHD or depression, if the neurotransmitter level is low, having more receptors or enhancing the sensitivity (turning up the volume) of these receptors can lead to a decrease in symptoms.

The female brain is sensitive to low-estrogen conditions (e.g. premenstrual, post-partum, and menopause) during which mood swings, irritability, sleep disturbances, and other cognitive problems are seen. It is these low-estrogen states that may present an added burden for girls and women with ADHD after puberty and menopause. The decreasing levels of estrogen seen at these times may result in a decreased sensitivity or lowering of the volume of the receptors in girls and women that are already compromised by lowered levels of transmitters (dopamine and/or serotonin) and/or by having smaller functioning brain areas (prefrontal and interconnecting sub-cortical areas). A worsening of the symptoms of ADHD, an increase in mood disorders, and impaired cognitive functioning may then be the result.

In 1990, Hans Huessy first addressed the issue of hormones and their relationship to ADHD by noting that girls with ADHD may have increasingly severe problems with the onset of puberty. He wrote that increased hormonal fluctuations throughout the phases of the menstrual cycle result in increased ADHD symptomatology.[32] In addition, more severe PMS including increased irritability and mood swings has been reported by adolescent girls with ADHD. Interestingly, anecdotal reports indicate that many women with ADHD can remain quite functional until they enter menopause, with its concomitant decrease in hormone levels, at which time, they no longer are able to cope as effectively with their ADHD symptoms. Despite these anecdotal reports, until we study girls and women with ADHD and the effects of puberty, menopause, and varying hormone levels, we may not have the answers to many of these questions.

INCREASING SYMPTOMS OF ADHD IN GIRLS AT PUBERTY

Puberty is a time of great turmoil and change. As the brain approaches maturity, it is exposed to a dramatic increase in adrenal hormones during adrenarche (awakening of the adrenal glands) and a year or two later, to an increase in sex hormones (testosterone and estradiol) during gonadarche (breast and genital development). These hormonal changes at puberty have long been blamed for the mood and behavior changes seen at this time. In studying a group of children who had premature adrenarche (turning on of the adrenal glands, but not sexual development), researchers were able to study the effect of hormones without the interference of social factors on behaviors. In this study, it was found that the children with earlier onset of puberty also had significantly higher levels of adrenal androgens, estradiol, and cortisol than children who began the process at the age-appropriate times. It was reported that the children with these higher-than-normal levels of hormones had significant psychosocial problems, including anxiety/depression, attention and behavior problems, impaired cognitive functioning, and poorer school performance.[33]

ADHD in most cases is present from birth, but for many girls the symptomatology of ADHD does not become bothersome until they reach puberty. A worsening of symptoms of ADHD may be seen at that time. In addition, a girl's impaired executive functioning may manifest only then as disorganization and performance worsen in response to life's increasing demands. Mothers of girls with ADHD report that their daughters experience a significant increase in irritability and mood swings starting at puberty. However, to date, no studies have been undertaken in girls with ADHD to determine if the worsening of symptoms they exhibit after puberty may be related to higher levels of adrenal and sex hormones or whether widely fluctuating hormone levels cause an actual worsening of ADHD symptoms and depressed mood at that time.

One study using fMRI was able to show the inefficiency of the prefrontal cortex (PFC) in girls with ADHD when compared to those without ADHD when given a working memory task.[34] An earlier study of younger girls with ADHD did not find as great a degree of executive dysfunction as in boys, but this may be a factor of the ages of the girls studied. The girls may have been too young to manifest the symptoms of brain dysfunction to the degree often seen after the onset of puberty.[35] Another study of adolescent girls found that brain dysfunction measured by reduced glucose metabolism was correlated with Tanner stage (the degree to which a girl had entered puberty as measured by breast and pubic hair changes). The further along the development of these secondary sexual characteristics, the greater was the brain dysfunction, regardless of the girl's chronological age.[36] This study has not been replicated, but it seems to report issues similar to those found in studies about the correlation and timing of psychological and behavioral disturbances in girls with higher than normal levels of hormones during puberty discussed earlier in this section.

CONCLUSIONS

What have we learned from all of this new information about the brain? First, that ADHD is a developmental, brain-based disorder most likely the result of various influences (including a genetic predisposition) on the brain during critical developmental periods before and after birth. During these times, the brain is most susceptible to injury and other insults that impact its development. ADHD is not the result of poor parenting, poverty, or other environmental causes.

Second, differences in the male versus female brain with ADHD exist and have been documented in both animal studies and in research including preschool and elementary school-aged children as well as adolescents. These differences most likely contribute to the symptoms of ADHD which affect a girl's behavior, academic achievement, and social functioning on a day-to-day basis and account for the differences seen in girls versus boys with ADHD. Third, and more importantly, as the brain approaches maturity, it is exposed to significant monthly hormonal bombardment uniquely affecting and complicating ADHD in girls. (We will discuss this further in later chapters.) Lastly, recent research has also demonstrated significant differences in structure and functioning in the brains of girls with ADHD when compared to girls without ADHD.

CHAPTER THREE

The Preschool Years
Little Girls with ADHD

THE PRESCHOOL YEARS ENCOMPASS that time from roughly three to five years of age when a girl develops a sense of self and begins the process of mastery, self-determination, and venturing out into the larger world. It is a time of intense exploration and explosive changes, both physically and emotionally, and the time when a girl acquires skills for beginning her academic career in elementary school. Diagnosing ADHD during this period can be difficult, but there is evidence that the diagnostic criteria used for ADHD can be applied to preschool-aged children. A review of the literature, including the multi-site study of the efficacy of methylphenidate in preschool-aged children,[1] revealed that the criteria could appropriately identify preschool children with ADHD. The accuracy of early childhood diagnosis is supported by a study showing that children diagnosed with ADHD between ages three and six years with a careful, thorough, multidisciplinary evaluation continue to meet diagnostic criteria several years later[2] – which is in marked contrast to recent articles suggesting that only half of children diagnosed with ADHD in preschool met criteria for ADHD several years later. Another recent study reports that among those children diagnosed early that no longer meet ADHD criteria a few years later, most continue to have problems with social and academic adjustment and demonstarte signs of other psychopathology.[3]

While diagnosis in this age group may be difficult, especially for those with predominantly inattentive symptoms, it is extremely important because when we can identify a girl with ADHD this early and provide appropriate treatment, we can increase her chances of succeeding in school and prevent problems with self-esteem in the future. The American Academy of Pediatrics recognizes the importance of early diagnosis and recommends that the primary care clinician initiate an evaluation for ADHD for any child four through 18 years of age who presents with academic or behavioral problems and symptoms of inattention, hyperactivity, or impulsivity.[4]

Children diagnosed with ADHD during this early developmental period usually stand out from other children because of their hyperactive behavior. However, by ages 6-7, inattention symptoms come into play and are somewhat superior at discriminating ADHD from non-ADHD children.[5] As a result, the majority of preschoolers diagnosed with ADHD are usually of the hyperactive or combined presentation. In one study of 50 preschoolers (25 with and 25 without ADHD), 68% were the hyperactive-impulsivity type, 28% combined type, and only 4% inattentive type.[6]

Disruptive behaviors and hyperactive/impulsive symptoms are more frequently observed among young children with ADHD than are inattentive symptoms. In the preschool-age group (12% of the children referred to a psychiatric clinic), the most common conditions identified were attention deficit hyperactivity disorder (86%), followed by disruptive disorder (61%), mood disorders (43%), and anxiety disorders (28%). Co-occurring psychiatric disorders were common among preschoolers, with most demonstrating two or more disorders.[7]

When you look at two groups of children diagnosed with ADHD, those in preschool (average age of onset just over 2) and those of school-age (average onset just under 4), a study reveals that the groups did not differ in symptoms of ADHD. Both groups had similar psychiatric coexisting conditions with over 70% of children in each group being diagnosed with other conditions. In addition, both groups were found to have substantial impairment in social, school, and overall functioning.[8]

Younger children with ADHD tend to exhibit higher activity levels than older children with ADHD, and their behaviors may be more situational. Behaviors also may not be as pervasive, and may occur more at home than at school. Mothers frequently blame themselves when their child acts out only at home. They feel that they cannot handle the situation and that they are the cause of the problem. Many feel that if they only had better parenting skills, things would be better. While counseling to improve parent-child relations does improve the situation, this does not mean that the parent was the cause of the problem. Frequently, we only see the problem at home when a girl is younger because this is the setting in which she is most comfortable being herself.

This does not mean that a real problem does not exist. Remember that true ADHD is a neurobiological condition and is not caused by poor parenting. Although poor parenting skills can make the problem worse, as we have seen, they are not the cause of the problem. Being a parent is a difficult and time-consuming job, at best. Being the parent of a daughter with special needs can be extremely challenging and frustrating, as well as exhausting.

Since one of the chief characteristics of this developmental stage is being active, how do we diagnose ADHD in preschoolers? According to research on this subject, it is the preschooler's quality and degree of activity that is the crucial factor in distinguishing her from normal, naturally energetic, and exuberant peers.[9] For those girls with hyperactivity at this stage, we often see more purposeless running and jumping, more up-and-away behaviors, and greater risk-taking involving climbing and other dangerous activities. As a result, these children often have more accidents, injuries, and emergency room visits.[10, 11] Difficult temperament as displayed by emotional reactivity was also found to be related to hyperactivity symptoms over time.[12]

In addition to activity level and emotional reactivity, other behavioral clues can be helpful in evaluating the significance of any disruptive or inappropriate behaviors in a preschool girl.

- Is she aggressive?
- Does she have difficulty with transitions?
- Does she engage and explore her environment or does she appear solitary or withdrawn?
- Do certain textures or types of clothing bother her?

- Does she have difficulty falling asleep or staying asleep?
- Is she difficult to console, or is her reaction out of proportion to a given situation?
- Are tantrums unprovoked?
- Does she crave movement?
- Does she engage in risk-taking or dangerous behaviors?
- Is she highly impulsive?
- Are there problems with eating or toileting?
- Is she excessively withdrawn?
- Can she follow directions?
- Does the normal oppositional behavior of the terrible twos continue as she becomes three, four, and beyond?
- Does she snore? Yes, snore! Enlarged tonsils and adenoids can cause sleep apnea and behavior disorders in young children and studies have shown that a simple adenoidectomy can significantly improve ADHD symptoms.[13]

With so many issues that can cause problems, how are parents to know if their daughter's behaviors warrant further investigation? In general, there are usually two behavioral patterns that predict an ADHD diagnosis. The first is preschool expulsion, usually resulting from aggressive behavior, refusal to participate in school activities, and/or failure to respect other children's property or boundaries. The second, peer rejection, is one that parents can easily identify. Children with extremely shy or bossy behaviors are often avoided by their classmates, ignored or shunned on the playground, and in other ways isolated or rejected.

While the previous questions and discussion may have left you concerned or questioning whether your daughter may have ADHD, they are not diagnostic for the disorder.

DIFFERENT PRESENTATIONS OF ADHD

While preschool girls with ADHD may have problems in each of these areas, they usually fall into one of two presentations designated in DSM-5 — the hyperactive/impulsive or the inattentive/distractible presentations. [14] Many of the girls found in this latter subgroup appear to be shy and withdrawn, in addition to inattentive and distractible. However, it should be noted that many girls demonstrate characteristics from both subgroups and don't fall into any clear pattern. No matter what subgroup a girl may fall into, the important issue is to identify her problem behaviors early to mitigate later academic, emotional, or social difficulties.

But how do we recognize ADHD girls as toddlers or preschoolers? Let's look at each presentation separately.

HYPERACTIVE/IMPULSIVE PRESENTATION

Jessica's mom knew early on that Jessica was different from her older sister. She had very advanced motor skills. She sat up early; she was pulling herself up at seven months and walking by nine months. She was always on the go and required little sleep. "Getting her to sleep at night and after nighttime feedings was very difficult. My husband spent hours rocking her on his shoulder." By age three, Jessica still wasn't sleeping through the night, and she had given up her daytime naps at 18 months. "She crawled out of her crib before she could walk and was always exploring or getting into things. While her running everywhere was appropriate as a young toddler, by age three we wanted more walking and less running."

Such girls may have trouble falling asleep at night or will wake up early in the morning. During these times, they frequently will get out of bed and play, or perhaps clean out their bedroom drawers, dumping all of the contents on the floor. In the morning, their rooms often are in disarray and they may be found sleeping on the floor, in a closet, or under the bed.

Hyperactive preschoolers may frequently engage in dangerous activities, including climbing. One eighteen-month-old was found on top of the dining room table, literally swinging from the chandelier and jumping off onto the dog's back as he ran around the table! Preschoolers with impulsive risk-taking behaviors also may stand out in other ways. Jamie's mom thought that Jamie was just accident-prone or perhaps more clumsy than other five-year-olds, but after her second broken bone and her third trip to the emergency room for stitches, Jamie's pediatrician questioned whether her risk-taking behaviors were out of the ordinary. In numerous studies, young children with ADHD have been described as more accident-prone. Of all behavior variables, it was the amount of general activity that was most strongly related to accident frequency.

In some girls with ADHD, hyperactivity may present as hyperverbal or hypertalkative behavior rather than as motor activities such as running or jumping.

> *Cathy talked early and her language development was precocious. However, she couldn't stop talking and commented on everything. While this appeared cute at first, it quickly became a problem for her peers and family members, who were often overwhelmed just trying to keep up. This type of chatter can be very disjointed and frequently off the topic of the conversation. "While everyone else was*

discussing what he or she wanted to order at the restaurant, Cathy was talking about why Ronald McDonald has a red nose or the present she wanted for her birthday." Such girls may ask a million questions or chatter on endlessly. More than one mother has been heard to remark, "I wish she would just stop talking for one minute. She even talks to herself nonstop while playing alone."

Other girls may be active, but engage in more age-appropriate and acceptable activities:

Lang liked to play outdoors and was very athletic. She loved to climb trees and preferred to play with boys, but not always in a dangerous way. She was very coordinated and rode a two-wheeled bike without training wheels by her fourth birthday. She was usually cooperative and had a good relationship with her father. He enjoyed her competitiveness and gutsy attitude. She could hit and throw a ball better than most boys her age, and was always sought after to play in their games.

Some girls at the hyperactive end of the ADHD continuum are strong-willed and controlling and may have problems when playing with peers. Aimee was one such girl. Her mother characterized the situation in the following words: "All games must be her idea and played by her rules. She assigns the roles each are to take when playing, and she is usually the mother!" This behavior also caused problems between mother and daughter since Aimee always wanted to be in control. The home situation for such girls frequently may be described as more intense than in other families. It has been observed that mothers of such children tend to talk and play less with them. Mothers are also more frustrated and may tend to use more physical punishment with these girls.

Teri was not only very hyperactive, she was also bossy, and control was a major issue for her. Problems arose around eating and toilet training, as she tried to remain in control of all situations. There were only a few foods that she would eat, and these were mainly eaten as she got up and down from the table a million times during a meal. She refused to go to the potty and started preschool in Pull-Ups®. As time progressed, her mother realized that Teri was too busy to stop and eat or use the potty. She also realized that these areas had become battlegrounds in the war for control. "In the end, I realized that the harder I pushed, or the more I yelled, the more firmly entrenched Teri became. Our days consisted of my yelling and Teri screaming or having one temper tantrum after another. My husband couldn't stand it. He blamed me for acting as bad as Teri. He said I was constantly getting down on her level and acting like a three-year-old myself. We argued a lot, but some days I couldn't disagree with his assessment of the situation. I didn't even like being around my own daughter."

INATTENTIVE/DISTRACTIBLE OR SHY/WITHDRAWN PRESENTATION

In the late 1960s, researchers at NIH studying a population of preschoolers found that some girls with ADHD presented behaviors that were the opposite of those expected — they were shy and withdrawn.[15]

Samantha is just such a preschooler. She had been a good baby, and was very placid and adaptable. She did not make great demands on her world as an infant. As she grew into a toddler, she did not readily join in with the other children, rather she watched from the sidelines. She tended to play by herself, overfocusing on one activity. She could play alone for hours when engaged in a favorite or familiar activity. However, when presented with multiple stimuli, she seemed overwhelmed and unable to focus on one thing. When given directions or tasks to perform, she tended to get distracted or lost along the way, playing with something else that caught her eye. At times, when sent on an errand, she would get to the destination, but then forget what she had been sent for. Too many directions at one time overwhelmed her and she frequently reacted like a deer caught in the headlights.

Other parents have referred to these daughters as, "my child who stops to smell the roses." Some girls may be thought to have language delays or auditory processing problems. Most parents and professionals rarely contemplate the diagnosis of ADHD, but, unless the diagnosis is entertained, these girls can be dismissed and overlooked for years. They sit in the back of the classroom not causing any trouble, but they have no idea what is going on because their minds are somewhere else. They are perceived as ditsy or not very smart, and many years are wasted as they grow to believe that they are not capable of achieving at the same level as others.

"Melinda began using a few words by the age of 18 months. Then at two years, she slowed down. As Melinda's world expanded into new experiences with nursery school, visits to the library and swim time at the local pool, I realized that not only did Melinda continue to stare at strangers; she invariably was the last to participate in an activity. While all of her friends were bustling and shoving to be first, she hung back, reluctant, gazing

out windows and smiling sweetly." Her mother took her for a speech and language evaluation as well as a hearing test. As expected, her hearing was normal, however, Melinda did demonstrate some difficulty with processing language, particularly when there was a lot of noise and commotion. She also had difficulty when she was given more than a single command. At the age of eight, Melinda was evaluated by a neuropsychologist who reported that she exhibited many characteristics of ADHD. But, because she was not hyperactive, her parents had great difficulty convincing both the school and medical personnel of the diagnosis.

SCHOOL READINESS AND ADHD BEHAVIORS

Behavior problems can have a significant impact on kindergarten readiness. Childhood behavior problems are associated with substantial delays in motor, language, play, school, and socioemotional skills. In one study, children with behavior problems were reported to enter kindergarten with lower speech and language, motor, play, and school skills, even after controlling for demographics and region. Parents of children with behavior problems were also five times more likely to report that their children were not ready for kindergarten.[16] For girls with ADHD, difficulties seen in school may also stem from inattentive or impulsive behaviors which result in inefficient cognitive styles. Early problems with cognitive control have been found to correlate with inattention and hyperactivity.[17] While no one girl may fall perfectly into a particular subtype, it has been shown that the problematic behaviors correlate with later academic competence and achievement. Studies of three-year-olds revealed a significant association between problem behaviors, poor rapport, and task orientation. Those preschoolers with behavior problems had a tendency to be more active and fidgety and to show extreme moodiness.[18] At age 3, overactivity in boys, and shyness and difficulty separating in girls, were shown to be correlated with behavior problems at school at age five.[19]

AUDITORY PROCESSING AND RECEPTIVE/EXPRESSIVE LANGUAGE SKILL DEVELOPMENT

Ability to follow directions and to process verbally-presented information (auditory processing) may be delayed in children with ADHD. In one large study,[20] language ability (as measured by receptive vocabulary) and mother-rated inattention-hyperactivity and externalizing behavior problems were measured biannually from ages four to 12 years. Results showed that language ability predicted later behavior problems more strongly than behavior problems predicted later language ability, suggesting that the direction of effect may be from language ability to behavior problems.

Children with ADHD may also have difficulty expressing themselves and/or have expressive language delays, which can affect their overall cognitive functioning. As one study documented, 3-year-old children with ADHD symptoms (reported by parents) and language delays (reported by their teachers) performed significantly worse than those with only ADHD symptoms on most language-related cognitive measures. There were no differences between the groups on most nonverbal measures.[21]

As a result of these additional language issues, preschoolers with ADHD may have difficulty paying attention, processing information, and answering questions about a story read to them.

They may also not be able to relate clearly what went on at home or during the day at school. For such girls, visual clues (pictures) can be used to help to orient them and provide a framework to organize their language. In addition, the need for sameness is essential to improve their ability to follow directions or know what to do next in a sequence of steps or routine activities.

ADHD, EARLY LITERACY, AND LATER LEARNING

Preschool problems of inattention, hyperactivity, and impulsivity impact the development of early literacy skills and broader school achievement in later years.[22] One study[23] of preschool children found that inattention affected emergent literacy skills while hyperactivity/impulsivity did not. In another study teacher ratings of attention-memory were found to predict word reading above and beyond the contribution of phonological awareness and vocabulary knowledge in a group of 432 kindergarten students.[24] The results of both of these studies show that inattention uniquely affects the development of early reading skills, placing young girls who experience problems with attention at greater risk for later academic difficulties.

ADHD AND EXECUTIVE FUNCTIONS IN PRESCHOOLERS

Preschool children with ADHD were also found to have problems with the executive functions (EF) relating to inhibition and working memory. Lack of inhibition in young children was found to be associated with ADHD, disruptive behavior disorders (DBD), and poorer working memory performance. Inhibition and working memory performance did improve over time, especially in the early preschool period in children with ADHD versus typically developing children.[25]

HOW DO GIRLS WHO ARE DIAGNOSED LATER WITH ADHD BEHAVE IN PRESCHOOL?

Let's look at how the typical girl with ADHD behaves in the preschool classroom, based on the DSM-5 presentations we have been discussing.

Hyperactive/impulsive girls in the classroom

The hyperactive and impulsive girls with ADHD usually can be easily spotted in the preschool classroom. They have a great deal of energy and engage in lots of movement around the room. They never stay with one activity or play with one toy for any extended length of time. They go from activity to activity, but never really engage. When seated activities are required these girls do not stay at the table for very long and show a considerable amount of up and away behavior. These girls tend to be bossy and more aggressive with other children. On the playground, they may engage in dangerous activities, such as scrambling to the highest rung on the climbing equipment, or into the branches of the tree which has been specified as off limits. They may wander away and tend to run from or ahead of the group. Field trips may be difficult, and these girls may need an adult assigned to just look after them.

In addition to having difficulty sitting still, hyperactive/ impulsive girls with ADHD may be talking, asking questions, or interrupting constantly. They like to dominate any situation, and they require a great deal of attention. Indeed, they seek to be the center of attention, and make it clear that they are not happy if they are not in that role. These girls are always seeking novel stimuli. However, when asked to recognize materials that have been presented before, they may act as if they have never seen them. They also tend to answer impulsively, giving fewer correct responses than their peers. They may demonstrate motor impulsivity, which also can be seen in their drawings. They tend to rush through craft activities, and draw much faster than other children. These behaviors present problems for establishing early learning patterns, and cause difficulty with tasks such as learning, numbers, colors, and letters.

Naptime may be particularly difficult, as these girls need little sleep. Having long ago given up their naps at home, they have difficulty staying still in one place. They may prefer to roam around the room, sing, or talk through nap or quiet time, becoming a general disruption to others.

Negative classroom behaviors

At school, initially, the girl with difficult behaviors may not display all of the behaviors observed at home. However, she will eventually have difficulty meeting the demands of her class work. Perhaps she will have trouble starting an activity, or she may not want to finish when time is up, or when others are done with this activity. Power struggles will gradually appear in this setting, as well. These girls may cry more often and be more negative in general. They will have difficulty if offered too many choices, and can't easily make up their minds. They are inconsistent. On some days they may not want to nap, while on other days they may actually sleep for long periods.

Reactions may be out of proportion to the event, and these girls frequently have difficulty controlling their reactions. Angry displays such as foot stomping, arms crossed over the chest, and biting may become issues in the classroom. These girls may misperceive the behaviors of others, feeling that they have been slighted, or feeling that their space has been invaded when no slight was intended. Their behaviors tend to escalate and these girls may need physical restraining or frequent time-outs away from the group in order to calm down. Moods and responses are unpredictable and change quickly. These girls may be perfectly delightful while on a field trip and only have difficulty when it's time to leave.

Inattentive or shy/withdrawn girls in the classroom

The girls who are shy and withdrawn may look very different from hyperactive/ impulsive girls in preschool. Their behaviors may isolate them from the other children, and they frequently may be seen observing the others from the sidelines of the group. They appear as daydreamers, and can be easily distracted from a task. They have difficulty transitioning from one task to another, and may always be one step behind the others. They frequently misplace or lose mittens, hats, coats, and even their shoes.

These girls often appear to prefer solitary play, and frequently overfocus on an activity. They become lost in what they are doing, and are unaware of what is going on around them. At times, they seem confused. Naptimes and clean-up times are difficult because of the transitions involved. These girls are not very adaptable, and have difficulty with new routines or personnel in the classroom. Field trips present problems because of the break in routine and the new surroundings.

Making the diagnosis of ADHD in preschoolers

Many of the behaviors described in this chapter are perfectly appropriate for toddlers up to the age of three. So how can you tell if there is a problem and that the behaviors you are seeing are more than developmental? Making a diagnosis of ADHD in children in this preschool period remains a controversial issue, but one that needs to be addressed if we are to avoid the negative effects on self-esteem, relationships, and academic potential that multiply as the years progress without a proper diagnosis.

If you are concerned about your preschool daughter, take her to a pediatrician, child psychologist, or child psychiatrist. Diagnosis of ADHD should involve a thorough medical and developmental history, observation of social and emotional circumstances at home, and feedback from teachers and health professionals who have contact with her. In many cases, other testing may be needed to rule out conditions, discussed previously, whose symptoms might overlap with ADHD, including anxiety disorder, language-processing disorders, oppositional-defiant disorders, and sensory integration problems.

SEEK THE HELP OF PROFESSIONALS

The most important first step toward obtaining a diagnosis is seeking the help of professionals trained in working with young children. While many professionals are well trained and have experience with elementary-school-aged boys, very few have experience or expertise in diagnosing preschoolers or girls.

Gathering information from preschool teachers, daycare providers, and babysitters also will be helpful. These professionals have experience in dealing with many children in this age group. If your child does not attend a preschool, you might consider placement in a qualified preschool program. Qualified preschool programs include programs such as Head Start or other public prekindergarten programs. If your other children did not have ADHD, it may be difficult for you to decide if there really is a problem. An experienced preschool teacher can be a great resource to help you sort out what is developmentally appropriate behavior.

ADHD is a diagnosis based on history and observed behaviors (symptoms). There is no specific test for ADHD, and the disorder cannot be ruled in or ruled out by looking at a child's behavior in only one setting. Ask questions and read as much as you can. Be aware that the diagnosis exists in preschoolers, and learn how it presents in girls. This is the only way that you will be able to ascertain if your daughter, student, or patient has ADHD.

GATHERING INFORMATION FROM OTHERS
THE USE OF RATING SCALES AND QUESTIONNAIRES

Using questionnaires and asking questions are the two best ways for gathering information to make a careful diagnosis of ADHD. Questions, such as the ones offered at the end of this chapter, may be very useful in alerting you to the possibility that there is a problem. However, an accurate interpretation of information obtained from multiple assessors is indispensable when making the complex diagnosis of behavioral problems in children. Be aware that parents and teachers don't always agree about children's behaviors.

In one study of kindergarten children with and without behavior problems, low levels of parent-teacher agreement were found on their overall ratings of the children's behavior with the greatest agreement seen on the rating of children without behavioral problems. However, parent and teacher ratings did correlate with the usual prevalence of ADHD in this population and seem to do so independently of each other. [26] Combining parent and teacher measures has been found to be an effective way to determine if a behavior issue exists.[27] Further confirming the importance of obtaining these ratings from several sources when attempting to make a diagnosis of ADHD.

Seek out early identification programs

All school systems must, by law, have programs to identify children at risk for behavior or learning problems. This is another avenue you may wish to pursue. Head Start and early identification programs in your area should offer screenings and evaluations. Preschool-aged children who display significant emotional or behavioral concerns might qualify for Early Childhood Special Education services through their local school districts. The evaluators for these programs and/or Early Childhood Special Education teachers will be excellent reporters of ADHD symptoms.

Gathering information from within the family

ADHD often runs in families.[28] Consider whether either parent has symptoms of ADHD, diagnosed or undiagnosed. If one or both parents have ADHD, there is a high likelihood that the children will, too. Siblings of children with ADHD have two to three times the risk of having ADHD compared to children who don't have siblings with ADHD. Talk with other family members. Has anyone else had the same problems as a child? Have other siblings, cousins, nephews, or nieces been diagnosed with ADHD or learning disorders?

Consult with your daughter's pediatrician

Talk with your daughter's pediatrician. He or she should be able to discuss her development up to this point and any risk factors related to the pregnancy and/or family history. A physical examination, vision and hearing tests, and developmental screening should be conducted when the diagnosis of ADHD is being considered. This testing can rule out other conditions that may be contributing to your daughter's behaviors. In addition, psychological testing will help rule out specific learning differences and aid in defining learning strengths.

However, because many pediatricians are not trained in the diagnosis of ADHD in children this young, it is important to convey your concerns and assess if they are being seriously addressed. Don't feel that your pediatrician has all the answers, or that you are being disloyal for seeking help elsewhere. It is still rare that a pediatrician recognizes ADHD, especially without hyperactivity, in a preschooler.

After the diagnosis

Once a preschool girl has been diagnosed with ADHD, there are several positive steps you can take to make things better at home and in preschool. The most important first step is seeking help. Girls with ADHD are more difficult to handle in many settings. Whether your daughter is hyperactive, shy, irritable, or stubborn, you and her teachers need to become aware of how to assist her in becoming better integrated into a preschool or daycare program, and that includes relating positively to others.

Parent behavior training (PBT)

When dealing with children less than six years old, research shows that parent behavior training (PBT) and emotion socialization programs designed specifically for hyperactive preschoolers, were highly effective in improving a child's behavior, even when compared to studies involving combined home and school/day care interventions, or methylphenidate use.[29]

It is important to read about ADHD and learn how to parent a difficult child. Attend parenting classes or seek the help of a therapist or family counselor to assist you. Learning new behavior management techniques is extremely important. They can help you better deal with your daughter's behaviors and address or eliminate problem situations such as transitions. Studies conducted over the last several years are consistently documenting the effectiveness of parent behavior training interventions, when compared to other interventions, including medication for treatment of preschoolers at risk for ADHD [30] One study in particular revealed that parents who took part in a 14-week parenting program that involved teaching parenting strategies for managing hyperactive and disruptive behavior, as well as emotion socialization strategies for improving children's emotion regulation, reported significantly less child inattention, hyperactivity, oppositional defiance, and emotional lability. These parents were also observed using significantly more positive and less negative parenting strategies.[31]

THE FOLLOWING ARE SOME TECHNIQUES YOU MIGHT TRY:

Remain positive

Parents, caretakers, and teachers need to remain positive. Remember it is the girl's behaviors that are the problem, not the girl herself. Many girls grow up feeling that they are bad, not very smart, or that there was something wrong with them because of the negative comments they've heard throughout their lives.

Choose appropriate activities

Working with an expert can help you choose appropriate activities for your daughter/student based on her developmental level. Appropriate activities can reduce her frustration and will help her build confidence.

Offer fewer choices

Girls with ADHD should be offered fewer choices to avoid power struggles and tantrums. If these behaviors do arise, they should be managed with firmness and consistency.

Use time-out

A brief time-out or simply ignoring the behavior may be appropriate ways to handle tantrums. Time-out works by removing the girl, who is out of control, from the situation and allowing her time to process and calm down. This technique, when used consistently and calmly, can be used with girls as young as two. The period of time-out should be kept brief and be used consistently with few words or explanations. The rule of thumb is one minute of time-out per year of age. The girl, herself, may even see the value in the practice and eventually may wish to put herself in time-out in order to gain self-control.

Holding

When a girl with ADHD is extremely out of control, or she is a danger to herself or others, the issue of holding often arises. Using this technique, the adult in charge of the situation will hold the girl tightly until she has calmed down. Girls often are able to tell you if they are okay or that they no longer need to be held. Time-out also may work if the girl is sufficiently in control at the time or once she has calmed down. Physical punishment or spanking is rarely appropriate under any circumstances.

Avoid power struggles

> As one mother put it, *"One of the most important lessons we have learned is the art of compromise. I have also had to learn to make a demand and wait when Carla is in one of her stubborn moods. Her overall goal is to please, but she has to reconcile how she can please me and not feel as though she has 'lost.' I usually give her a choice and then back off, so she can decide to do the right thing."*
>
> *"We had been using time-out at home for some time. Initially, when Mary's behaviors were out of control, we would*

consistently remove her to time-out. Over several months, she became used to it. Eventually, all I needed to say was, 'I think you need a time-out now,' and she would go over to a little bench we had set up in the family room, sit down, and look at one of her books. When she came back to the situation, she was usually calmer and more cooperative. One day, when I was visiting her nursery school class, I noticed that Mary was becoming excited during a game of musical chairs. She was laughing and starting to touch and pull on the other children. I could see things escalating and getting out of control. All at once, Mary ran from the group, sat in a big beanbag chair, and held up a book to cover her face. I was amazed. She was giving herself a time-out, just like at home. After a few minutes, she seemed calm and rejoined the group when invited. I was so proud of her and glad we had been using the technique at home."

Anticipate and plan

In working with a girl with ADHD, it is also important to anticipate difficult situations. Difficult situations may include transitioning to bed, meal-time, toilet-training, playing with others, and getting along with siblings.

DEALING WITH DIFFICULT SITUATIONS

Bedtime

Bedtime may precipitate many problem behaviors. For some girls, bedtime represents a time of separation from parents or older siblings. This issue needs to be addressed with understanding and consistency. Bedtime rituals, firm limit setting, and constant reassurance are usually enough to address this problem. Allowing a child to stay up until she is tired or ready for bed does not address the issue, and usually results only in a tired and cranky child the next day. Many children demand that their parents remain in the room or lie down with them until they fall asleep. Some prefer to fall asleep in the parents' bed or come into the parents' bed during the night. Neither of these solutions addresses the issue of separation or control, and is therefore not adequate. For girls who need little sleep, playing quietly in their room or listening to tapes of music or stories may be an option.

> *"I now recognize that Keisha just does not need as much sleep as her older sister. I allow her to stay up later and play in her room until I come up and turn out the light. Putting her in her own room has helped because now we are not worried that she will wake her older sister or baby brother. We also bought her a set of headphones and she loves to listen quietly to music or stories on tape. These also work great on long car rides."*

For girls who awaken and get up during the night, it is important to offer protection from dangerous situations, such as going outdoors alone, climbing on high objects, or getting into the kitchen near the stove, etc. This may be accomplished by locking the kitchen door, setting up a gate in the bedroom doorway, or double-locking the front door of the house. Alarm systems are now relatively inexpensive and can be set up with motion detectors and an alarm that sounds when a door or window is opened. Bright girls with ADHD are very creative. Parents just need to be more creative in finding solutions.

> *"Jessica had started waking up very early, before 6 AM on the weekends. Gone were the days when she would entertain herself in her room, playing and looking at her toys. She would get up, go downstairs, eat food, and make*

a mess. After a string of what I thought were impossible days, one when she had climbed up on a chair, opened the freezer, gotten out ice cream, left the freezer open and gone out on the back deck to eat the ice cream, we decided we needed to do something. My husband sawed her bedroom door in half (like an old 'Dutch' door) and we put a lock on the bottom half. When Jessica was safely in her room and had been kissed good night, we locked the bottom half. We repeated, as she had been told previously, that if she needed us, all she had to do was call, and that in the morning she could have a 'treat' with breakfast if she stayed in her room. It worked like a charm, and we felt better knowing that Jessica was safe!"

Toilet-training

Toilet-training can become an area for confrontation and power struggles. In general, girls are trained more easily and are developmentally ready sooner than boys. However, if a girl is not ready, she should be allowed more time. If wetting occurs because of lack of awareness, frequent reminders or scheduled visits to the bathroom may help. Early accidents as a result of not paying attention to the need to go to the bathroom are common. However, they can lead to embarrassment and cause a girl to not want to leave home. Bedwetting is seen more frequently in children with ADHD and may be an issue for girls as well. Handling this situation with caring and concern is the best approach.

"Toilet-training had been late for her sister, so I was not worried when Jessica started preschool in Pull-Ups®. As time progressed, however, I realized that she used Pull-Ups® because it was convenient; and she did not have to stop what she was doing to go to the bathroom. I put her in underwear and told her she would earn a sticker every

time she used the potty. Within a week, she was happy and no longer even asking for stickers. Bowel movements have been more difficult, but again, the stickers worked very well. The last hurdle will be to not wear Pull-Ups® to bed."

Mealtime

Control issues and behavior problems also may arise around mealtime. Some girls have difficulty stopping an activity in order to eat. Others may have issues with food textures and preferences. It's best to deal with sensory issues with an occupational therapist, as part of a total treatment program for sensory sensitivity. Control and attention issues need to be addressed separately, with limit setting and a behavior management system — a system that rewards appropriate behaviors, such as tasting a variety of foods or eating small amounts of a non-preferred food, with an extra serving of a preferred food.

"By the time Carrie was three, she would only eat macaroni and cheese, applesauce, and yogurt. I was concerned about her nutrition, and when our pediatrician told me after a check-up that she was slightly anemic, I was really worried. Because of some other sensory hypersensitivity (Carrie didn't like labels on her shirts and would only wear soft sweat pants), he recommended we see an occupational therapist. She explained to me about problems with hypersensitivity, and we began a program to gradually increase what Carrie would eat. It took several months, but by being consistent and offering her rewards and her favorite foods as treats, we gradually added to the foods that she would eat. She eventually started eating hamburger, soups with chicken and vegetables (cut up in small pieces and puréed at first), and other mashed fruits. We continued occupational therapy

and a desensitization program. Eventually, the pieces of food she could tolerate became larger."

Remember Teri and her mother from earlier in this chapter? They were also having difficulty in the area of control around toilet-training and mealtime. Well, their story also has a happy ending.

"With the help of our family therapist, I set up a behavior program to address these issues with Teri. I decided to pick one behavior and try to focus on changing it rather than constantly trying to change everything at once. I chose getting up from the table before she had finished her food as the behavior to target. It was difficult, but with constant reminders and smaller portions, she gradually could eat a meal at one sitting. From here, we moved on to going into the bathroom and sitting on the toilet. I realized these were small steps, but we were now making progress."

Social interactions

Playing with others, such as siblings or peers, also can be a problem area. Rough play may lead to over-stimulation and problems with stopping an activity. Play dates with only one or two other children may need to be arranged. Planned, supervised activities usually work out better than unsupervised or unstructured playtimes. The child with ADHD needs to know the limits. Acceptable, as well as unacceptable, behaviors should be reviewed beforehand. Large gatherings such as birthday parties can be difficult, and behaviors usually deteriorate as excitement escalates. Planning a smaller get-together is usually more successful. Girls who are shy and attentive also may find large groups overwhelming.

"When participating in preschool birthday parties in the neighborhood, Melissa always seemed overwhelmed.

Instead of showing excitement by plowing into the games and candy like the other children, she would cling to me and refuse to get off my lap or unwrap herself from my leg. She would smile, but refuse to take her goody bag, and seemed on the verge of tears the rest of the time. Other mothers commented on her distress, and I was worried that she would soon not be invited at all. I was also dreading her birthday in the fall. When that time came, we decided just to invite another quiet little boy and girl, who were her friends. We set up a video in the family room and had cake and ice cream without singing 'Happy Birthday.' Her friends only stayed for about an hour and all seemed to go well. Melissa even seemed genuinely unhappy that they were leaving when it was over."

Girls with ADHD may have difficulty interacting with older or younger siblings. Play with younger siblings may need to be supervised as a young girl with ADHD may have difficulty controlling her enthusiasm or impulses. Often, they may also irritate older siblings by invading their space or tagging along. It is important that off-limit areas (such as older siblings' bedrooms) be set up and strictly enforced. It is important to also try to avoid always assigning the role of babysitter to older siblings. This may cause them to resent their little sister. However, older siblings may be called into service occasionally on a contractual basis, once they are old enough to understand how to properly supervise and deal with their younger sister with ADHD in a helpful way.

CHOOSING THE BEST PRESCHOOL

If you are looking for a preschool for your daughter for her first school experience, or if your daughter is having difficulty in her current preschool placement and you are thinking about making a change to another environment, there are several things you need to consider to ensure that your daughter's school experience will be a success.

Don't just look at the school

Choose a school that is the best match for your daughter's needs. While reputation, location, convenience, price, and values are important, it's critical that instead of looking for the best preschool, you look for the best match ***for your daughter***. They may be two different things! Make sure you speak to the administrators and teachers to get a better understanding of their approach to learning and how they specifically approach the child with ADHD. What do they offer? How do they position these children for success? Classroom placement within a school is also important.

HERE ARE SOME THINGS TO LOOK FOR

Smaller classrooms with less stimulation and a strong routine

This can often make a tremendous difference in improving ADHD symptoms in preschoolers. Schools that work well for children with ADHD, tend to focus on structure and consistency as core foundations to learning. Structure and support will also help your daughter know what to expect from the environment and what is expected of her in return. Classrooms, as well as home, should be childproofed to protect the impulsive preschool girl.

Best teacher match

Girls with ADHD do better in a structured setting, but it is always important to seek out as good a match between teacher and student as possible. Teachers are role models for your daughter. Teachers who are impatient or judgmental will make most kids averse to learning. The teacher's attitude and education regarding learning differences, the school's philosophy, and individual teaching styles all need to be taken into consideration. You want your child to be taught by people who are firm but offer integrity, and who create a safe and comfortable learning environment.

Support for all developmental skills areas

Placement should take into account the individual needs of each girl. This includes such issues as activity level, disorganization, fine and gross motor development, and need for structure and creativity. Make sure that the school has access to a team of experts to help insure your child with ADHD is getting all of the support she needs to be successful.

Hands on approach to learning

Children with ADHD do better with a hands-on approach. Look for a school where your child will be actively engaged in learning and not be asked to sit and listen for hours. Regularly scheduled exercise is also important.

Be an advocate

Many parents don't have the flexibility to choose the school that their child will attend. If that is the case, your most important role is to know your daughter and to advocate for what she needs. You'll want to be on the same team as the teachers and administrators at your daughter's school and work together to maintain a dialogue to ensure success. Be sure that you have open and free communication with your daughter's classroom teachers, and request all of the school's resources available to help your daughter.

TREATING ADHD SYMPTOMS WITH MEDICATION IN PRESCHOOLERS

The Preschool ADHD Treatment Study, or PATS, conducted by the National Institute of Mental Health (NIMH), is the first long-term study designed to evaluate the effectiveness of treating preschoolers with ADHD with behavioral therapy, and then, in some cases, methylphenidate, a stimulant for the treatment of ADHD. In the first stage, the children (303 preschoolers with severe ADHD, between the ages of three and five) and their parents participated in a 10-week behavioral therapy course. For one third of the children, ADHD symptoms improved so dramatically with behavior therapy alone that they did not progress to the ADHD medication phase of the study.

Only those children with the most severe ADHD symptoms, who did not improve after the behavioral therapy course and whose parents agreed to have them treated with medication, were included in the medication study. In the first part of the medication study, the children took a range of doses from a total of 3.75 mg to 22.5 mg of methylphenidate per day, administered in three equal doses. (By comparison, doses for school-aged children usually range from 15 to 50 mg total daily.) The study then compared the effectiveness of methylphenidate to placebo and found that the children taking methylphenidate had a more marked reduction of their ADHD symptoms compared to children taking a placebo, and that different children responded best to different doses. The study also found that while preschoolers with ADHD may need only a low dose of methylphenidate initially, a higher dose may be needed later to maintain the drug's effectiveness. Mild side effects were noted with a decrease in height and weight from expected values reported. Eighty-nine percent (89%) of the children tolerated the drug well, but 11% had to drop out of the study as a result of side effects. Other side effects included insomnia, loss of appetite, mood disturbances such as feeling nervous or worried, and skin-picking behaviors.[16]

For girls with a high level of hyperactivity or impulsivity, or who are dangerous to themselves or others, the use of medication, even at this young age, may be indicated. Aggressiveness and uncontrolled temper tantrums may negatively affect family and/or peer relationships, and for these girls the use of medication can be a lifesaver. The stimulants and other medications used to treat these disorders are discussed in more detail in Chapter Eleven.

OTHER THERAPIES AND TRAINING

Additional therapies may be necessary to address motor or language delays. The girl with ADHD may already be experiencing learning difficulties based on her cognitive style; the additional burden of other developmental delays may further complicate the situation. An occupational or physical therapist and/or a speech pathologist may be necessary as adjuncts to her educational program to deal with language delays, hypersensitivities or sensory integration dysfunction, and fine or gross motor coordination difficulties or delays. Placement in special education or programs for children at-risk for learning difficulties may be appropriate in order to avoid problems in the future.

In addition, programs that enhance executive, attention, and motor skills have been found to be useful even in the preschool population. In one study,[17] the authors recruited parents to engage regularly with their preschool child in a series of games that enhance inhibitory control, working memory, attention, visuospatial abilities, planning and motor skills. Parents played with their child for 30-45 minutes/day and taught strategies to enhance these skills. This program included such games as *Simon Says* and *Freeze Dance,* or remembering shopping lists or the location of treasures hidden under cups. After the five to 10 weeks of sessions and games, significant reductions in both parent and teacher ratings of ADHD symptoms were reported as determined by pre- and post-treatment testing. In addition, the results continued to be observed at one and three month follow-ups with the parents reporting continued game times, although fewer per week and of a shorter duration on average by three months.

CONCLUSION

One of the most consistent characteristics of ADHD is its inconsistency. Coupling that with the normalcy of some of these characteristically ADHD-behaviors before the age of three makes ADHD difficult to diagnose in the preschool years. Having said this, however, it is imperative that we begin to do a better job of diagnosing ADHD in preschool populations. The early diagnosis of ADHD is important for several reasons. Early diagnosis leads to earlier access to treatment and intervention programs; such early intervention programs can prevent many secondary problems from developing. Early diagnosis allows for the establishment of good habits and patterns, sets up positive relationships, and encourages the development of better parenting skills. Your daughter will also feel better about herself.

In this chapter, we have discussed several separate presentations of ADHD in girls of this age group. But, life is rarely so simple or clear cut. Your daughter, student, or patient may be displaying symptoms of both inattention and hyperactive/impulsive subtypes of ADHD. Diagnosticians have also observed this phenomenon, and have resolved this issue by designating a combined presentation of the disorder.

In addition, we have presented some other symptoms that manifest in these early years. We need to look at shy/withdrawn preschoolers and better document their difficulties within the subgroup of the inattentive/distractible girls with ADHD. And what of the girl whose early problems don't result in academic difficulties until later elementary years or middle school? What of the young girl, who has frequent mood swings, is overly sensitive, or who cries often and easily? Does she later go on to have depression as well as ADHD? As of yet, we don't have answers to all of these questions.

However, there is much that we can do to help girls with ADHD live happier, more satisfying lives, and the sooner we start the better. Preschool is ***not*** too early. Much of the damage to self-esteem and interpersonal relationships is already well under way by the age of seven. If you feel that your daughter or student is experiencing difficulty, seek an evaluation or professional guidance. You and she will be glad that you did.

QUESTIONS TO ASK YOURSELF ABOUT YOUR PRESCHOOL DAUGHTER

This list was designed to raise your level of awareness and aid you in asking the right questions. We encourage you to take a look at your preschool-aged daughter, student, or patient with these typical behaviors in mind, and to seek further evaluation if your suspicions are aroused by the following questions.

- Is she restless or overactive?
- Does she run instead of walk?
- Does she have trouble sitting still?
- Is she always up and on-the-go?
- Is she squirmy and fidgety?
- Does she have a short attention span? (10-15 minutes is average for this age.)
- Does she have difficulty concentrating on or playing with one toy for any length of time?
- Does she have difficulty listening to a story being read to her?
- Does she engage in dangerous activities?
- Does she not show appropriate fear?
- Does she have frequent accidents (stitches, cuts, bruises, broken bones, or visits to the ER)?
- Does she bully other children?
- Is she bossy?
- Does she kick, bite, or hit others?
- Does she have difficulty sharing toys?
- Does she often stare into space?
- Is she a daydreamer?
- Does she give up easily?
- Does she often stand on the sidelines and watch before joining in a group activity?

- Does she worry excessively?
- Does she prefer to play on her own (solitary play)?
- Is she fearful or afraid of new situations?
- Does she speak very little in public?
- Does she have delayed speech or language skills?
- Does she have difficulty expressing herself?
- Does she misplace or lose belongings?
- Is she irritable?
- Is she miserable or unhappy?
- Does she cry often and easily?
- Does she have temper tantrums?
- Is she fussy or overly particular?
- Does she blame others?
- Do others like her?
- Does she destroy toys?
- Is her toilet training delayed (beyond three years)?
- Does she still wet or soil herself, although she's trained?
- Does she rarely nap or rest quietly, even when tired?

CHAPTER FOUR

The Elementary School Years
What's Normal and What's ADHD?

TO BEST APPRECIATE THE SPECIAL challenges faced by elementary school girls with ADHD, it is helpful to view them against the backdrop of typical development for this age group. In most cultures, after age five, children are no longer restricted to the home or to settings where they are closely monitored by caregivers. Instead, these young children are challenged to become increasingly responsible for their own behavior in a variety of new social contexts. To succeed within this framework of greater autonomy, elementary school age children are expected to gradually take over some of the responsibilities that have previously been the domain of adults. Many children begin to learn to plan ahead, prioritize, organize, and monitor their own behavior during this stage of development. Beginning in infancy, but clustered during the elementary school years, the skills that compose the executive functions emerge.[1]

One of the defining developmental characteristics of this stage is greatly increased cognitive capabilities — the ability to think logically and flexibly, to keep track of more than one thing at a time, to perform tasks independently, to formulate goals and resist the temptation to abandon them. Jean Piaget believed that the key to these increased cognitive capacities lay in the crystallization of a higher form of thought that he called concrete operations. This new level of reasoning enables children to make their physical world more comprehensible and predictable. For example, when children understand that they can pour water from a tall pitcher into a short bowl and the volume of water remains unchanged, they can begin to think more flexibly, and make better approximations and predictions about the future. Each discovery affords them more control over their world, and allows them to venture forth with more confidence.[2]

As they begin the process of separating from their parents and home environments, elementary school girls can become freer to focus their energies on school challenges, both academic and interpersonal. School begins to occupy a central role in their lives, and provides an abundance of new stimuli from teachers and peers. The skills necessary to process all of this new information are being learned continuously throughout this period. As young girls play together, usually in pairs, they interact in a pretend or fantasy context in which they can engage in complex verbal negotiations. This play-acting helps them to understand much about the give-and-take necessary for successful communication.[3]

It is during this time that the girls who exhibit behaviors that are not in keeping with these developmental expectations may be noticed. At one end of the ADHD continuum are the inattentive girls who may be observed at the fringes of peer groups, processing information slowly, already missing some jokes, and not keeping up with the quick repartee of other girls. Since language deficits seem to occur more frequently among ADHD girls vs. boys, [4] these inattentive girls are beginning their social development at a disadvantage. At the other end of the continuum are the girls who demonstrate hyperactive and/or disruptive behaviors. These more impulsive girls experience difficulty fitting in to the typical social interactions of elementary school aged girls because they are less able to pay close attention to the verbal and non-verbal communications of the girls around them. They may impulsively interrupt and may demand that things be done their way rather than compromising in order to maintain the social relationships with other girls. Because these girls are often more disruptive, they are the most likely to be referred for assessment.[5]

As these girls broaden their focus to school and beyond, interacting with peers, teachers and other adults, they enter into the long-term task of developing an identity beyond their role within the intimate family circle. One of the most critical roles that parents (and other adults) can play during these formative years is to help shield girls with ADHD from a relentless stream of negative reactions and criticisms, so that their identity development is not permeated with negative self-images.

It is important to remember that throughout elementary school development is notoriously uneven — both in terms of the chronological appearance of skills within a given child, as well as between children across a given skill. In the face of constant changes in emerging abilities, it is not surprising that adults can forget that even dramatic developmental differences are normal. The realities of uneven development can be quite anxiety provoking for the parents of girls with ADHD, who witness their daughters struggling with skills that have been mastered by the majority of their peers.

To make matters more confusing, even though most elementary school girls with ADHD experience these difficulties to varying degrees, the way their symptoms are expressed can differ greatly. The following classifications of behaviors are based on the descriptions of ADHD presentations outlined in the DSM-5.[6] We use them here primarily for convention, since it has been shown that these presentations do not remain stable over time.[7] Nonetheless, the three classifications serve to highlight the heterogeneous exhibition of ADHD symptoms in elementary school girls.

THE PREDOMINANTLY HYPERACTIVE/IMPULSIVE PRESENTATION

> *When I was called in to evaluate Jan in first grade, her teacher voiced concern that Jan simply could not sit still at circle time, despite various and repeated interventions. She said that the other children found her behavior annoying and intrusive, and were reluctant to sit next to her. The teacher, Mrs. Leeds, felt that Jan was bright and understood what was expected. She didn't find Jan to typically be oppositional, but was at a loss to explain her behavior. When I was alone with Jan, I shared the teacher's concern. She responded, "I know Mrs. Leeds wants me to sit still. I want to sit still. Every day, I tell my tushie to stay in my spot in the circle, but it doesn't listen to me."*

Jan's statement poignantly captures the conundrum inherent in having one's behavior defy one's intentions. Sadly, Jan's behavior did cause children to avoid her, and she rarely was invited for a play date. However, in the long run, Jan may have been lucky that her hyperactivity was so pronounced. Despite the fact that she was smart enough to mask her other ADHD symptoms, her physical symptoms were intrusive enough that she came to her teacher's attention. Eventually, she was referred for evaluation and diagnosed at an early age.

> *In a typical scenario, Debbie raced two boys to the school bus, and shoved her way through the line to make sure she won the race. As she moved toward the back of the bus, she felt someone kick her. Debbie felt pain, humiliation and, above all, anger. She lashed out before she could even think. Debbie never considered that perhaps this was an accidental incident on the chaotic and overcrowded bus. She gave no thought to the probability that her punch would be seen by the bus driver and reported to the principal. She had no idea that there could be a non-aggressive solution to the situation, and she was oblivious to the likelihood that her peers would reject her because of her aggressive response. Even though Debbie violently punched the boy she believed to be the culprit, she was still angry as she got off the bus. On her way off, she impulsively banged her backpack into several other children, loudly announcing that everyone on the bus was a bunch of losers. Later, the boy's mother called Debbie's mother to discuss the incident. When her mother brought it up, Debbie, who was no longer angry, burst into tears and said, "It wasn't my fault."*

Elementary school girls like Jan and Debbie, whose most overt symptoms are characterized by hyperactivity and impulsivity, are easily identified because their behaviors appear similar to those of boys with ADHD. These girls are recognized because their behavior is not appropriate, especially relative to society's gender role expectations. These girls have been shown to have more problematic peer relationships and more externalizing symptoms than the combined or inattentive girls.[8] Even today, with less emphasis on traditional gender roles than ever before, girls with ADHD who behave like boys with ADHD face severe consequences. Indeed, it has been shown that the most hyperactive girls, who are also physically aggressive, are at the greatest risk for a variety of future psychological adjustment problems.[9] As hyperactive/impulsive symptoms typically decline, this presentation becomes increasingly less visible with age.[10]

THE COMBINED PRESENTATION

This presentation of ADHD combines hyperactive, impulsive, and inattentive symptoms. For girls with combined presentation ADHD, their hyper behaviors are more gender typical, such as being animated and talkative, while their distractibility interferes with attention to the task at hand. A typical scenario follows:

> *Rachel is in her fourth grade math class, whispering enthusiastically to the girl next to her. The increasingly louder chatting attracts the interest of the girl behind her, too. Feeling very much the center of attention, Rachel begins making some sort of proclamation, and she bangs her desk with her pencil for emphasis. She loses her grip on the pencil and it goes flying two seats away. The boy who picks it up is engaged by Rachel's mischievous mood and won't give her pencil back to her. Giggling hysterically now, Rachel gets out of her seat and goes over to demand*

her pencil. The teacher immediately addresses her, and Rachel says, "Well, I can't do my work without my pencil." Rachel laughs, the other children giggle nervously, and the teacher asks Rachel to see her after class.

Rachel's behavior, while disruptive and impulsive, is not angry or aggressive. The Rachels of this world may be seen by parents and teachers as silly, as having chutzpah, or as being obsessed with the drama of their social lives. Although not as troublesome as hyperactive/impulsive girls, families with combined presentation children experience more adversity than families with inattentive presentation children. The problems reported by the parents of these combined presentation girls related more to ADHD symptoms of inattention and disorganization than to conduct problems.[11] It has been found that, for combined presentation girls like Rachel, their math skills decline over time, compared to girls without ADHD, whose skills improve with age.[12] Because math skills are cumulative, this may be a reflection of not attending and truly mastering earlier math skills upon which more advanced math skills depend. The intellect of combined presentation girls is likely to be underestimated, and their underlying issues are often masked. As we will soon see, girls who don't manifest hyperactivity are not necessarily lucky.

THE PREDOMINANTLY INATTENTIVE PRESENTATION

Girls with an inattentive presentation may constitute the majority of girls with ADHD.[13] However, because their symptoms are more subtle and less easily observable, they are the girls who are most likely to be mislabeled, misunderstood, or overlooked completely. Because their symptoms are more internal and difficult to observe, self-report scales (like the one at the end of this book) are particularly important to diagnosis, allowing girls to report internal experiences that may not be apparent to parents and teachers. Even young girls can acknowledge feelings that they might not have volunteered without the prompt of a questionnaire.

More passive and less direct than the combined presentation girls, their behaviors are more in keeping with standard notions of femininity. Since they tend to internalize their symptoms, they bring much less notice to themselves in the classroom; far from being disruptive, they dread being the center of attention. Fearful of criticism, they are generally cooperative and compliant, hoping to win their teacher's approval. However, they rarely feel confident about their knowledge and tend to avoid class participation. They process information slowly, and may speak haltingly in class, with awkward silences. They have difficulty following multistep directions and completing classroom assignments on time. They often daydream in class, and benefit from an attuned teacher who will touch them lightly on the shoulder to discreetly refocus them, rather than startle them by calling out their name. Despite disorganized desks and messy backpacks, these girls are often described as sweet and shy by their teachers, who may not recognize the subtle signs of ADHD struggles in these girls. In fact, inattentive girls have significantly more academic difficulties than inattentive boys, including less academic motivation, lower academic expectations, lower GPAs and lower IQs.[14]

The dilemmas that Carly encounters in her fourth grade classroom are all too typical for an inattentive girl with ADHD:

> *When Carly wakes up, she tells her mother she has a headache, and doesn't think she can go to school. Her mother urges her to go anyway, although she knows that Carly*

desperately wants to stay home. When Carly arrives at school, she has trouble with her locker combination, and gets to class a few minutes late, feeling self-conscious and ashamed. Mrs. Barton is discussing "Charlotte's Web," which the class has been reading for the past few weeks. Carly quickly gets to her seat in the back of the room, next to the tank holding two geckos. She is often pleasantly distracted by their skittering about and today is no exception. On days like today, she feels trapped like the geckos, and imagines being free to be outside. She dreads being called on by Mrs. Barton, and wishes she were invisible; she looks down so that they don't make eye contact. Carly is behind in her reading. As is typical for her, she starts out motivated to read, gets about 20 pages in, and then starts to lose interest. It becomes harder and harder for her to stay focused, which causes her to reread the same pages over and over. She hasn't even looked at the book in a week, and she feels like everyone in the class knows it. It's in her locker, so she couldn't get it out anyway.

Now Mrs. Barton tells them to choose a partner to discuss an alternate ending for the current chapter. Carly's stomach begins roiling as soon as she hears the word 'partner' and, as she watches the others pair off, her eyes are holding back tears. No one ever chooses to partner with her; she is usually left to work with Bruce, the other student no one likes. Carly is painfully shy, and waits for Bruce to speak to her, but he's busy seeing how far back he can tilt his chair. They are silent when Mrs. Barton comes to intervene. Carly didn't really hear the assignment because she was so upset, but she is afraid to ask Mrs. Barton to repeat it. Mrs. Barton asks Carly to start off the discussion with Bruce, and Carly looks at her blankly. Mrs. Barton often feels that Carly is just not paying attention, and she is clearly annoyed that she has to start the conversation for them. After Mrs. Barton provides some direction, she walks away. Carly meekly suggests a vague idea, and Bruce tells her it's stupid, just like she is. Tears begin to run down Carly's face.

Socially, inattentive girls fare worse than inattentive boys in terms of both peer relationships and self-concept. These girls have been found to be significantly less popular and more likely to be bullied.[15] Because of their social isolation and peer rejection, these are the girls who cry quietly into their pillows, but insist to their parents that nothing is wrong. Girls with ADHD are more likely to experience significant internalizing symptoms than either boys with ADHD or girls without ADHD.[16, 17] The longer the diagnosis of ADHD is delayed, the more the symptoms of psychological stress increase, which, in turn, increases the likelihood of adjustment problems in adolescence.

In elementary school girls, their secondary symptoms of anxiety and depression are just beginning and rarely reach the level of a true disorder. Still, with their clear difficulties in the academic and social realms, it is not surprising that the inattentive girls are more likely to have a coexisting anxiety disorder than boys with ADHD, and should be monitored carefully.[18]

GIRLS WITH A HIGH IQ

It's the super-smart girl with predominantly inattentive presentation of ADHD who is least likely to be diagnosed in a timely manner. The smarter she is, the more easily she can coast through the elementary years without exhibiting overt symptoms. Her high grades convince people that there's nothing wrong. Her intelligence allows her to easily compensate for her difficulties, leading her teachers to ignore some odd or shy behaviors. And, the more she succeeds, the more pressure there is for her to continue to seem smart. One study found that the gifted children who had also been identified as having ADHD were more impaired than other children with ADHD.[19] This may suggest that the superior abilities of these gifted children can mask ADHD symptoms to varying extents, and that there may be many gifted children with ADHD whose ability to compensate makes them less likely to be diagnosed. In fact, one study of gifted students found that nearly 10% of them qualified for an ADHD diagnosis, though none had been identified.[20]

It has been reported that the social and emotional development of children with ADHD lags about three years behind their same-age peers.[21] This is equally true for gifted children, who have even greater discrepancies as their intellectual abilities may be three years ahead of their peers. This six-year discrepancy between their intellectual capacity and their emotional maturity can be daunting for the gifted child, or her parent or teacher to make sense of. In fact, it has been shown that having superior intellectual abilities and ADHD may result in social and emotional factors that produce a heightened sense of anxiety, overreaction, and peer rejection.[22]

Because their symptoms are, for the most part, invisible at this age, these girls can use their superior intellect to help them compensate. They may be able to mask their chronic difficulties with disorganization, lateness, and forgetfulness in school. The report cards of these smart and inattentive girls will assure their parents that their daughters are sweet, quiet, bright, but perhaps not working up to their potential. It is only at home that they can let down their defenses and be seen for the daydreamers they are. In fact, these high IQ girls have been found to have more coexisting mood, anxiety, and disruptive disorders than ADHD girls with average IQs. This study suggests that the internalized anxiety of these smart girls may reduce disruptive behaviors that would otherwise alert others to the possibility of ADHD.[23] This dynamic may be yet another factor that inadvertently serves to keep the struggles of gifted girls with ADHD hidden.

PERFECTIONIST / OBSESSIVE TENDENCIES

Parents and teachers alike need to learn to recognize the possible underlying problems for girls who may appear to try too hard to succeed. Just as for girls in general, girls with ADHD keenly feel the societal pressure to be neat, organized, and well behaved.[24] One common way of managing their difficulties is to develop rigid perfectionist tendencies that help them hyperfocus in order to get their work done. Their achievements are not without cost, as success involves significant struggle.

> *It's Sunday night at 9:00 PM. Valerie, a third grader, is about to go to bed when she looks at her diorama, due tomorrow, and thinks the teacher will like the project better if it has an attractive sign on the front. Feeling pressured to finish quickly, she cuts out a rectangle from a blue sheet of paper she finds on her floor, not noticing that there is a school permission slip for parents on the other side that will never make it to her parents. She alternately trims a tiny strip off one side and then the other, trying to get the sides to be perfectly straight, until the paper is much*

smaller than she had intended. She prints the title, which seems insignificant on the small paper, so she decides to embellish each letter with a design.

Valerie is completely engaged in repeating the design carefully on each letter when her mother calls to remind her that it is past her bedtime. Valerie says she'll be done in a minute. However, she didn't look ahead and the design, which got increasingly bigger with each successive letter, resulted in the last letter running over the edge of the paper. Frustrated, she erased furiously, wrinkling the paper, and rewrote the letter, pressing so hard that the pencil point broke. Now, with a newly sharpened pencil, she retraces the new letter until the paper tears through in one spot. She is angry at herself for tearing the paper, and is looking for a new piece of paper when her mother comes in, annoyed that Valerie is still up. Valerie is ashamed to show her mother the ruined sign, and just tells her she's almost done. Her mother says it's too late to do any more work, and that Valerie needs to learn that there are consequences for forgetting to do her work. Valerie argues that "it's not fair," but her mother insists that Valerie get into bed. Valerie bursts into tears, and her mother is terribly conflicted about how to handle the situation. Valerie is sure the teacher will hate her project, and that everyone will make fun of her sign.

For Valerie, obsessive tendencies are a way of compensating for the ADHD tendency to overlook details; often, these girls with ADHD feel they must force themselves to attend to every detail in response to societal expectations that females have it all together, and be neat, as well.

HOW ADHD INCONSISTENCY COMPLICATES THE ELEMENTARY SCHOOL YEARS

Parents of girls with ADHD are predictably perplexed by the fact that their daughters' perform inconsistently. This *consistent inconsistency* is hard to accept and hard to comprehend. Parents can understandably be seduced when they see flashes of the higher cognitive understanding they hope for in their daughters with ADHD. Buoyed by witnessing a new level of functioning, they raise their overall expectations accordingly. These young girls try to comply, eager to earn positive feedback. However, the varying conditions that permit the executive functions to work together one day and not the next are not within their control. Parents may feel chagrined when their daughters seem unable to learn from their mistakes; they rarely alter their behavior and instead repeat versions of the same mistakes over and over again.

Learning to generalize from a specific situation to similar situations is a necessity for problem-solving in life. However, for girls with ADHD, the novelty of a situation can derail the fragile mastery of generalization that they have achieved. In fact, it has been shown that elementary school girls with ADHD have more trouble with planning and response inhibition than boys with ADHD.[25] Girls with ADHD are extremely reliant on routine and structure and, even when parents try to anticipate the challenges their daughters might encounter, small changes can easily make the familiar unfamiliar. When these girls fall short of previous accomplishments, it distresses all concerned.

> *Michelle is an 8-year-old girl with ADHD who joined the Brownies. Since this is her first extracurricular group activity, she finds their Tuesday afternoon outings both scary and exciting. Her troop sometimes returns from their local outings earlier than expected, and the girls are*

free to play until their parents arrive. Without structure from their leader, Michelle becomes overexcited and then upset. Parents are expected at 5:00 PM, but Michelle becomes increasingly impatient and is often crying by the time her mother arrives. Her mother solved this problem by having Michelle call her as soon as they return to the community center, and she does her best to pick Michelle up immediately. This plan was successful on two consecutive occasions, and both mother and daughter were pleased with the results.

When the troop went to the nature preserve, they took a minibus instead of walking, and the bus returned them to the elementary school instead of the community center. Michelle was confused, but she waited with the several remaining girls, trying not to cry. As the last girls were picked up, Michelle became frantic, not understanding why her mother wasn't there. At 5:00 PM, her mother arrived at the community center and was redirected to the school. When she arrived at 5:07 PM, Michelle was clinging to the leader, crying hysterically. When Michelle calmed down a half-hour later, she announced that she was going to drop out of the Brownies. As her mother tried to reason with her, Michelle put her fingers in her ears and sang loudly. Her mother felt guilty and offered to buy Michelle a new Beanie Baby.™ Michelle accepted the offering, but reminded her mother that she still would not return to the Brownies.

Just enough variables had changed to rob Michelle of her sense of control. Michelle often struggles with emotional dysregulation. Her strong emotions overwhelm her ability to think clearly and respond appropriately. It is thought that this tendency may contribute significantly to the social difficulties common to girls with ADHD.[26] Reacting with the emotional intensity frequently seen in girls with ADHD, she felt frightened and overwhelmed, and was no longer able to reason with clarity. This scenario reflects one of the most frustrating and frequent elements of parenting daughters with ADHD. Mothers teach their daughters a skill; their daughters demonstrate that they have learned the skill, but later instances arise in which they do not use the skill. Often, both mother and daughter are at a loss to explain why, and both feel frustrated and disappointed. Mothers may feel guilty for having unreasonable expectations of their daughters, while the daughters feeling guilty for having failed their mothers. Because the mother-daughter connection is so important, the temporary disruption of their relationship can evoke shame and even anxiety that go well beyond the simple failure to utilize a skill.

THE CHALLENGES OF CONNECTEDNESS

Carol Gilligan highlighted the gender differences between girls' and boys' definitions of moral behavior. Girls generally define morality in terms of conflicting responsibilities rather than the more male-valued terms of competing rights. In other words, a girl may feel that winning a game also leaves her opponent feeling sad, and she may perceive those as conflicting outcomes that may create anxiety for her. The comfort level of the relationship between the friends may have greater importance to her than her own achievement, which threatens to place her above her friend and disrupt their mutuality. On the other hand, a boy may be thrilled to be the winner, feeling that he has worked to earn his superior position over his opponents, as long as he knows he has played by the rules.[27] Gilligan uses the metaphors of the web versus the ladder to illustrate the distinction between girls' and boys' relationships. For girls, the web can symbolize interconnectedness; for boys, the ladder suggests hierarchical, achievement-oriented relationships.

For girls, ADHD-related impairments in social skills can prove to be particularly destructive, due to the more intimate nature of their social milieu.[28] Girls may sometimes make choices in order to maintain relationships, even when they interfere with their personal development. However, in contrast to these other-oriented choices, sometimes the impulse-driven behaviors of many girls occur before she is able to think of the possible consequences to her relationships with other girls. Girls with ADHD can pursue short-term goals with an intense hyperfocus, similar to the achievement-oriented behaviors more typical of boys. When they are so intently engaged, they may be perceived as selfish, bossy, or controlling. It is difficult for them to distinguish between what seems urgent to them versus what may be important to their peers. It may appear that these girls prefer competition over cooperation. However, they simply may be responding to the impulse of the moment, unable to focus on the feelings of peers at the same time.

Girls that are caught up in their impulsive, self-centered focus may experience peer rejection without understanding why. Indeed, girls with ADHD are more disliked by their peers than boys with ADHD, and are viewed by parents and teachers as substantially behind their non-ADHD peers in social development.[29] Repeated experiences like these can result in a growing sense of insecurity for girls with ADHD, steeped in the sense that they can't really trust their judgment because it so often betrays them.

Girls with ADHD engage in more socially awkward and problematic behaviors than girls without ADHD.[30] They are, in general, more aggressive than their non-ADHD peers. Specifically, the combined presentation girls have been found to be more aggressive than the inattentive girls, who are more aggressive than their non-ADHD peers. Girls with and without ADHD were found to dislike girls who exhibited any kind of aggression.[31] In one study, the more impulsive girls with ADHD were perceived as aggressive and rated very negatively by their peers, and the more inattentive girls were seen as socially isolated.[32] Being viewed by peers in either of these ways has a high potential for damaging the fragile sense of self of these girls.

One of the ways in which this social blindness may be manifested is through relational aggression. Because girls place such high value on social acceptance and emotional intimacy, harming the victim's relationships with others is a particularly effective means of manipulation.[33] Girls with ADHD may feel a sense of social control when using tactics that compel others to meet their needs. In some cases, relational aggression is indirect and involves planning and verbal skill (e.g. creating and spreading an elaborate lie) while, in other cases it is direct and involves intense impulsivity (angrily disinviting someone to a party). Researchers continue to tease apart the factors that contribute to these girls' tendencies toward relational aggression, but it is already clear that our understanding of the aggressive behaviors of girls with ADHD is central to appreciating their far-reaching social impairments.[34, 35]

SELF-ESTEEM

In general, a history of positive interactions contributes to the development of better self-esteem. Interestingly, despite experiencing consistent social failures, elementary school girls with ADHD significantly over-rate their social competence compared to objective measures or adult ratings. This positive illusory bias was highest for the more oppositional girls, and lower for girls with more depressive symptoms, but always higher than for girls without ADHD. The tendency to describe themselves in such a positive light may reflect the bravado typical of a defensive coping style, attempting to conceal their shame, and/or an inability to accurately assess their performance.[36] Equally of concern is the fact that the parents and teachers of girls with ADHD rated their academic performance as significantly more negative than is evidenced by objective measures. This distortion was greater for girls with ADHD than for elementary age boys with ADHD or for girls without ADHD.[37] While researchers continue to tease apart why girls with ADHD receive such negative assessments from parents, teachers, and peers, we do know that these negative messages become internalized.

Girls with ADHD in elementary school have difficulty making and maintaining friendships. In general, they tend to have few friends; inattentive girls may become overly dependent on one friend, and more impulsive girls may not be able to maintain any friendships. Even though the friendships of girls with ADHD have positive qualities similar to those of girls without ADHD, the ADHD relationships are also fraught with conflict and interpersonal aggression. When they do initiate a friendship, girls with ADHD tend to befriend other girls with ADHD, although those relationships are not described as satisfying.[38] Lacking the verbal and attentional skills necessary to share experiences or participate in conversations that aren't about themselves, they often receive negative feedback from their peer group, which can result in feeling lonely and isolated.

In a first grade art class, Marnie wants to color in the sky on her picture and needs a blue marker, but they are all being used at that moment. She demands loudly of the class, "Who's got the blue?" When children say they are still using the blue markers, Marnie throws a tantrum. She stamps her feet and insists, "I HAVE to do the sky NOW!" She runs up to two of the children using blue markers and grabs the markers out of their hands, leaving blue lines across their palms. She grasps both markers and goes back to color the sky with one marker, while holding the other tightly in her hand. Her classmates complain, and the teacher approaches, but Marnie does not give up the markers without a fight. She explains to the teacher, "I needed the blue more than they did." When the teacher explains why Marnie's behavior was unacceptable, Marnie cries and says she understands. Marnie joins her class at lunch, and gives each of the injured parties some of her lunch money.

Emotional neediness or her desperate desire to feel in control may indeed underlie Marnie's behavior. However, children and adults are likely to misinterpret this behavior. Because her impulses compel her to attend only to her own feelings, young girls with ADHD like Marnie are often described as rude, bossy, selfish, or mean.

When young girls with ADHD suddenly find themselves overwhelmed with stimulation, not even they can account for their inappropriate behavior. Such an ambush occurred while a third-grade class was rehearsing for the spring concert.

Melissa barely noticed that her one good friend, Cathy, had bumped into her because she was focused on singing, which she loved, and on keeping her balance on the bleachers. When Cathy, who stood next to her, bumped into her a second time, Melissa was annoyed for a few moments, but they were coming up to her favorite part of the song and she was able to refocus on her singing. When Louis stumbled on the bleachers and knocked into Melissa, Melissa assumed it was Cathy bugging her again. Suddenly, she felt intensely resentful and vengeful; without thinking, Melissa shoved the unsuspecting Cathy off the end of the bleachers. Cathy cried, the singing stopped, and Melissa was as shocked as anyone else. Her teacher asked why she had pushed her friend and Melissa answered honestly, "I don't know." This response annoyed the teacher and Melissa was sent to the principal's office, where she cried inconsolably. Because Melissa and Cathy often had play dates together, Melissa's mother was at a loss when the principal called to report the incident. Lately, Melissa's mother had begun to dread when the phone rang after school; it seemed that often a parent or teacher was calling to complain about Melissa's behavior.

In this case, Melissa was overstimulated by the cumulative effects of a wide variety of factors: the excitement of performing, the focus on making sure she sang her part when the teacher pointed to her side of the bleachers, and the general challenge of staying on the bleachers without falling. Needless to say, Melissa had no idea that she was near her limits of frustration tolerance and stimulation overload. When Louis bumped into her, it was the straw that broke the camel's back. Irritable from managing multiple demands on her sensitive sensory system, she struck out in a burst of discomfort.

This classic experience of being ambushed — by their own feelings or by the reactions of someone else — is central to the sense of feeling that their lives are out of control. Experiences with others seem random and unpredictable. That being the case, it is easy to understand why so many girls with ADHD withdraw from interactions rather than experience incomprehensible interactions that end badly. These examples illustrate the essential nature of the ability to monitor one's own behavior consistently — one of the critical developmental tasks that is delayed in girls with ADHD.

In a different type of self-monitoring failure, girls with ADHD can become so focused on their own experiences that they may find themselves ambushed by the responses of others.

> *Penny began to braid the hair of Mary Ann, who sits in front of her in class. Initially, Mary Ann accepted this and thanked Penny. However, armed with this positive reinforcement, Penny's spirits soared as she kept undoing the braid and re-braiding it. Soon, Mary Ann asked Penny to stop. Penny, giddy because she was connecting with another child in a seemingly intimate way, didn't really process the request. If anything, there was generally higher stimulation in Mary Ann's more intense response. Mary Ann became increasingly annoyed with Penny, until she finally turned around and yelled, "Don't touch my hair anymore!" Penny, feeling unexpectedly assaulted by Mary Ann's reaction, started to cry.*
>
> *Since she was unable to appreciate her impact on Mary Ann, she was shocked by Mary Ann's negative response, which seemed to come out of nowhere. It is easy to see that Penny has yet to achieve the developmental skills that would allow her to simultaneously monitor her own experience as well as Mary Ann's. As a result, she is unable*

to make the chaotic world of social interactions any more predictable for herself at this point in time. She learns that one of the risks of relationships is a painful emotional ambush.

These are daunting lessons that, over time, take a toll on the way these girls measure their worth in the world. A young girl with ADHD who says she's sorry she was born, or that there's nothing worth living for, should be taken seriously. Some parents may assume that these comments are simply dramatic or manipulative, misunderstanding the intensity of emotion in their daughter. Feelings of anxiety and depression can begin to develop during elementary school years in response to their interpersonal struggles. Intense feelings of unhappiness, combined with the impulsivity of ADHD, should be seen as red flags prompting immediate evaluation by a professional. Without intervention, there is a high likelihood that these emotional tendencies could develop into mood disorders by young adulthood [39] which, in turn, can increase the risk for further negative outcomes.[40]

THE ROLE OF THE FAMILY

It has been well-established that ADHD is a highly heritable condition, with genetics underlying the neurobiological symptoms.[41] The biological traits that a girl with ADHD is born with are strongly influenced by her social/psychological environment, especially that of her family. Family interactions influence the severity and overall developmental course of the disorder for better or worse.[42] It has been shown that parents of girls with ADHD feel more overwhelmed by their parenting role than parents of girls without ADHD.[43] An analysis of 44 studies confirmed that parents of children with ADHD experience more parenting stress than parents of non-ADHD children. Parental stress levels may be exacerbated by conduct problems in their child with ADHD as well as by parental depression.[44] One study explored the impact of the emotional environment of the home on elementary school girls with ADHD. They measured a criticism factor, which taps into parental feelings of hostility or resentment toward their daughters, and an emotional over-involvement factor, which measures self-sacrificing or over-protective attitudes. In these families, there was a strong tendency for parents to be both critical and intrusive, with high levels of expressed emotion (as they vacillated between frustration and anxiety in response to their daughter's behaviors. High levels of mothers' expressed emotion occurred in response to their daughters' ADHD symptoms, regardless of subtype. In other words, mothers are just as ambivalent and enmeshed with their inattentive daughters with ADHD as with daughters that demonstrated aggressive and/or oppositional behaviors.[45] These findings highlight the ambivalent, over-involved and sometimes toxic mother-daughter relationships that begin to form at this point in development.

Compared with girls without ADHD, girls with ADHD are more likely to be diagnosed with oppositional defiant disorder (ODD) and conduct disorder (CD).[46,47] When these girls do manifest externalizing behaviors, they tend to be more covert, such as stealing or lying, rather than overt behaviors like physical altercations, which are more typical of boys.[48] However, it is possible that it is the gender inappropriateness of their behaviors that are triggers for the negativity expressed by their parents. Parental negativity toward daughters with ADHD occurred even when no conduct problems were reported.

Because ADHD is familial,[49] there is a high likelihood that some of the parents of these girls also have ADHD and may struggle with impulse control themselves. Indeed, when faced with girls with ADHD who do demonstrate physically aggressive or openly defiant behaviors more typical of boys, some highly distressed parents, with impulsivity challenges of their own, resort to emotional and physical abuse. This possibility is supported by findings that girls with ADHD were more likely to have experienced physical and sexual abuse than non-ADHD girls.[50]

Despite the fact that many of the expressions of ADHD symptoms in girls evoke frustration and disappointment in their parents, there are many strategies to lower the emotional temperature of the interactions and instead strengthen a loving connection between parents and their ADHD daughters. There are a variety of interventions, such as counseling, coaching, cognitive-behavioral training, social skills groups, and medication that can help to extend a safety net beneath these girls as parents find their own strategies that can be successful for all. As we learn more about the unique clinical course and psychosocial needs of girls with ADHD, it becomes increasingly clear that interventions that are tailored to girls may be particularly helpful.

ADHD-FRIENDLY RECOMMENDATIONS FOR PARENTS

Structure home life

There are many concrete changes that can be made to help girls with ADHD play to their strengths. The overarching goal is to help them experience the sense of security and control that comes from living within the context of a predictable structure. This can be accomplished by instituting overt daily routines for the whole family to follow, including on the weekends. While these girls may say that they want to be left alone to do what they desire, an outline of expectations will actually contribute to increased focus. The greatest success will be achieved if the routines are arrived at jointly with your daughter; she will feel empowered by the opportunity for input. Parents can demonstrate their respect for her opinions by allowing her to make choices — from two options that you have pre-approved. For example, you can say, "Dinner is at 6:00 PM; would you like to shower before or after?"

Maintain realistic expectations

It is appropriate to expect most girls of this age to have some simple home responsibilities or chores. Often, a very explicit chart cataloguing these jobs can help keep them on track, especially if they are alternating jobs with a sibling. These charts can short-circuit a lot of the quibbling that can occur around expectations. The charts become even more effective if used in collaboration with a reward system. It can be helpful if chores are done at a routine time, daily, when a parent is present to remind and supervise. Again, the tone of the expectation should be a firm guideline without being rigid. For example, they can choose when, within a half-hour range, they want to take out the garbage. Help them develop a reminder system to keep track of their responsibilities and avoid last minute crises; transfer as much responsibility to them as is realistic. Your flexibility implies your respect for her, which makes it even more likely that she will take ownership of her responsibilities, as well as take pride in her accomplishments.

Although it is sometimes unclear whether they can't or won't perform a task, many loving parents are so attuned to their daughters' struggles that they anticipate the tasks that will cause their daughters frustration. Parents will perform these tasks for their disorganized and resistant daughters, hoping to protect them from painful experiences. For example, many parents continue to dress their dawdling 2nd graders in the morning in order to make sure they'll make the bus, and rush to find the Uggs^{tm} if their daughters reject the sneakers. They brush their 4th grade daughter's long hair and put it in a ponytail for them, while their daughters hurl instructions and complaints. Parents frantically rush to school with completed homework sheets that their 5th grade daughters left on the floor.

The problem with this approach is that it communicates an unspoken message: "I do this for you, because you can't do it for yourself." When parents correct the homework so that their daughters hand in a perfect paper, their teachers never get to know the real functioning of these girls and how they might best meet their needs. In addition, these girls learn that their work is not good enough unless their parents fix it first. They do internalize the message and begin to doubt themselves. If there is no clear expectation that they learn to master these skills, their expectations are shaped by these interactions — they don't even try.

As they mature, these girls become more dependent on their parents' interventions, while other girls are practicing the skills necessary for greater independence. Their neurologically delayed development becomes even further delayed, at the hands of empathetic and protective parents who only mean well. It is much more useful to give these girls the message that they can do these tasks. Praise their attempts to solve these problems and allow them to experience the consequences of failing. Parents can repeatedly underscore the importance of always trying your best, and express their praise for their daughter'seffort and their belief in her ability to succeed.

Remember that their brains need a break

After these girls expend monumental amounts of psychic energy holding themselves together throughout the school day, they need a break from the task of controlling their impulses. Ideally, home is the safe place where they can 'melt down' without negative consequences. It helps explain why many mothers notice that their daughters' behavior is worse after school than at other times. It's not that their impulsive behavior is targeted toward the parent, but that they feel secure enough to relax their defenses with the parents' protection.

After school is not the best time to ask about their day; while parents may desire to know, it's not the girls' best time to share. This period of time should be used as they choose, to shift gears, allowing them to regroup forces and adjust to the transition of being at home. It is helpful to explicitly label this as a predictable cooling off time, when nothing will be demanded, allowing them to engage in more passive activities, such as watching TV, playing a video game, or listening to music. This time should be part of the after-school routine, and everyone should be on the same page about when this respite ends and homework begins.

Increase the likelihood of social success

Many girls desire play dates after school without realizing that they no longer have the energy to tolerate more intense interactions at this time. In fact, without some downtime, many play dates turn into overstimulating disasters of demands and complaints. A structured after-school activity, carefully supervised, with a prescribed beginning and ending time, is often the most successful social context for these girls. When they do have play dates, they should be short, with a pre-arranged activity that might be best managed at your home, where a parent can monitor the signs of impending overstimulation. Unstructured and open-ended play dates allow impulses free reign. Parents come to retrieve their daughter, and a friendly chat can add another half hour when the girls have no activity, and don't know if the visit is over or not. For girls with ADHD, this confusing scenario doesn't allow them to know what is going to transpire. For parents who are in control, it's hard to remember how off-balance these girls can feel in the absence of explicit explanations.

For girls with ADHD, myriad opportunities for social networking exist on the internet, many of which are difficult for parents to monitor. For many girls, the anonymity emboldens them to try on new behaviors, in a context that they perceive to be judgment-free. Unfortunately, girls with ADHD are often bullied online by peers whom they know, as well as by those that pick up on their awkward social skills and may see them as easily victimized. In addition, the sexual curiosity of elementary school girls is easily pursued online and at parties. Parents should put their discomfort and disbelief aside; do not make the mistake of thinking that these issues do not affect elementary school girls. Music and videos convey highly stimulating scenarios that are especially tempting to the ADHD brain.

Exercise — a secret weapon

Exercise is an excellent outlet for all girls with ADHD. Studies find that regular exercise provides beneficial results in multiple realms. It can ameliorate symptoms associated with stress, anxiety, depressed mood, impulsivity, and negativity.[51] Exercise helps channel their restless energy, and provides physical challenges that increase focus. A healthy level of activity can shorten the time it takes them to fall asleep at night, and can improve the quality of their sleep. In addition, the endorphins released by the brain during aerobic exercise can elevate mood, just at the time of day when irritability may set in. After school is a good time to schedule exercise, whether it is bicycle riding, dance, or an organized sport. While it is important not to overload them with activities and stimulation after school, exercise can help release the tensions of the day, better preparing them to focus on homework later.

Keep sight of the big picture

Above all, parents should focus on treasuring the creativity, spontaneity, and energy that create the unique ideas that their daughters may consider. Make it clear that you are available to talk, but tolerate the fact that communication will flow most freely on their terms. Remind them (and yourself) that you are both on the same team, and keep your sense of humor. Create a foundation of trust so that they will be willing to expose their vulnerabilities to you. Elementary school issues are just the tip of the iceberg; these girls will be moving into middle school, where the greater sophistication of insight and cognition combines with the wild cards of puberty and sexuality to create complex problems without easy solutions. Developing healthy routines, supporting self-esteem, and modeling good communication will help prepare these girls to enter the high risk/high stress zone of middle school.

CONCLUSION

Elementary school may be the first time that girls with ADHD present with difficulties. If we are to change the course of ADHD and prevent secondary emotional, social, and academic issues from developing, it is important to intervene as early as possible. Many parents mistakenly reason that if there daughter is doing well in elementary school with their help at home that other interventions are unnecessary. Nothing could be further from the truth. Keep in mind that low self-esteem develops early and the foundation for other disorders is laid during these first critical years in school. Prevention of these difficulties and learning to live well despite ADHD depends on early diagnosis and treatment. Parents may need to become advocates for their daughter to make this happen.

QUESTIONS TO ASK YOURSELF ABOUT YOUR ELEMENTARY SCHOOL DAUGHTER

This list is designed to aid parents who may wonder about the possibility of ADHD in their young daughters. We ask you to consider your daughter with these questions in mind. Keep in mind that some primarily inattentive girls may hide their symptoms at this age, but may exhibit more obvious signs of ADHD when they are older. It is also important to understand that the development of different abilities progresses unevenly during the elementary school years, and that some concerning behaviors may disappear with time. Even if you answer "Yes" to many of the following questions, it does not necessarily indicate that your daughter has ADHD. However, if your concern is aroused, it may be advisable to seek the advice of a professional.

- Does she daydream frequently?
- Does she have trouble getting started on her home work?
- Is she easily distracted from mundane activities?
- Does she have trouble remembering multistep instructions?
- Does she seem resistant to reading for pleasure?
- Does she seem oversensitive and easily embarrassed?
- Is she generally disorganized?
- Does she struggle to get up in the morning?
- Does she often have a physical complaint (headache or stomachache)?
- Is she often late for school or other activities?
- Does she march to the beat of a different drummer?
- Does she usually stay up past her bedtime?
- Does she often lose or misplace items?

- Does she stay at the fringe of a large group activity?
- Does she sometimes wait until the last minute to go to the bathroom?
- Does she wish she had more friends?
- Does she often lose track of the time?
- Does she tend to be shy with other children?
- Does she seem forgetful or absentminded?
- Does she leave a trail of belongings throughout the house?
- Does she have a low frustration tolerance?
- Does she tend to interrupt conversations?
- Does she prefer to play with younger children?
- Does her teacher say she should speak up in class and try harder?
- Does she quickly become annoyed or irritable?
- Does she seem to overreact?
- Does she tend to put things off until later?
- Does she often seem as if she's not listening when you speak to her?
- Does she tend to blame others rather than accept responsibility?
- Is she thrown off by transitions?
- Is she often defiant and argumentative?
- Is she accident prone?
- Is she a very active tomboy?
- Is she a nonstop talker?
- Does she frequently interrupt?
- Does she have temper tantrums?

CHAPTER FIVE

The Middle School Years
New Challenges

WHEN YOUR DAUGHTERS WITH ADHD reach middle school, it is comforting to know that development is on their side. As they mature, they will have increasingly sophisticated cognitive abilities at their disposal to help override their impulses. If they have been hyperactive, they will likely become less overtly so, especially on the gross-motor scale.[1] Some of their symptoms will likely become less conspicuous and unwieldy, and thus more socially acceptable (which is not to say that the symptoms become milder, less pervasive, or less intrusive from the viewpoint of affected girls). Some of the overdue developmental steps discussed in the last chapter, such as self-monitoring, delaying gratification, transitioning, and generalizing, are likely to become more reliable during this period.

However, it is also likely that middle school daughters with ADHD will continue to lag behind their peers socially and academically, while their physical and intellectual development advances appropriately. As girls with ADHD progress into middle school, executive dysfunction becomes more apparent as demands upon them shift from a primary focus on self-regulation to more self-guided completion of heavier workloads, longer term assignments, and the organization of complex social demands.[2] Since girls present with the inattentive type of ADHD more often than boys,[3] and since they are not disruptive in class,[4] it is often this executive dysfunction that allows them to finally come to the attention of their teachers. As a result, there is a significant increase in the number of predominantly inattentive girls referred for evaluation at this age.[5]

At any cost, middle school girls want to conform. Regardless of the degree to which they struggle, it may be even more important for them to reject the idea of having a disorder or disability. Girls who were diagnosed in elementary school may begin to reject school accommodations, medication, or therapy. Girls who are referred for evaluation in middle school may fiercely deny the possibility of ADHD, claiming that there is "nothing wrong with me" and that there is "no way I'm like those obnoxious, hyper boys." Hormonal fluctuations undermine the stability of the latency stage of elementary school, unleashing intense and mercurial emotions that spark confusion and conflict within them.[6] Lacking validation from peers, their increasingly fragile self-esteem puts them at greater risk for psychological distress than boys with ADHD and girls without ADHD.[7, 8, 9]

This distress can exacerbate their ADHD symptoms and make the disorder more complex to treat. This unique set of potential risks for girls with ADHD merits consistent attention and intervention in order to avoid negative outcomes.

THE DEVELOPMENTAL CHALLENGE

Erik Erikson was one of many theorists who believed that establishing one's identity is the central task of adolescence. The early stages of identity development involve gaining an understanding of one's self and one's relationship with others. As middle school children begin to negotiate the processes of separation and individuation, they grapple with the demands of increasing autonomy. At the same time, they are working toward deeper and more complex relationships with peers. Finding a balance between becoming a separate individual and remaining connected to others is one of the greatest developmental challenges of this time.[10] However, even within the context of these universal developmental processes, the experience of girls diverges from that of boys.

GENDER ROLE EXPECTATIONS

In 1991, Shortchanging Girls, Shortchanging America: A Call to Action was the largest study of children and self-esteem. They found that, as girls approached adolescence, they lost confidence in themselves and their abilities. Most shocking was that a similar burgeoning sense of personal inadequacy was not experienced by boys.[11] Research has demonstrated that our society's gender role expectations can confound the already monumental undertaking of identity development for girls.

Girls traditionally rely on closer, more intimate social networks than boys, with greater levels of attachment and commitment. Unspoken rules dictate that girls favor peer connections over personal autonomy. While boys see themselves as autonomous beings, girls decline opportunities saying, "I can't, because my friend will feel bad if I do" (go without them, etc.). In other words, for middle school girls, there is virtually no decision made without taking their relationships into account. As a result, peer interactions become powerful determinants of self-worth for middle school girls.[12]

THE RELATIONAL PERSPECTIVE

For girls, psychological crises stem from disconnections, whether it is the beginning of normative separations from their parents, or the risks of asserting themselves before a jury of their peers. Societal expectations dictate compliance, passivity, and cooperation as the ideals of femininity, and girls soon learn that disagreement and opposition can drive others away.[13] Carol Gilligan explained that girls approaching adolescence often disavow their feelings and suppress their opinions in order to preserve relationships. Many girls conclude that the trade-off is worthwhile if they can avert rejection. As a result, they begin to silence themselves in an effort to remain connected, even to the point of abandoning their own voice. Although healthy relationships require mutuality, girls are willing to sacrifice their voice, rather than risk open conflict that might lead to isolation and rejection.

Winnicott theorized that the *true self* is free to develop when it is safe to be spontaneous, authentic, and uncensored—which is the context of early childhood for many girls. However, middle school ushers in the peak period of conformity to peer behaviors and beliefs. Girls dread peer criticism and fear that their *true self* will not be accepted. As a result, many girls begin to hide their *true self* in favor of a *false self* that they believe will better meet peer expectations.[14] After repeatedly silencing themselves, their creative insights and alternative scenarios are relegated to internal dialogues, and it becomes easier and easier to function with the *false self* in the lead. As a society, we are deprived of the voices of so many valuable girls whose ideas sit latent behind these façades.

ADHD AND IDENTITY DEVELOPMENT

These unfortunate developmental trends are only intensified for girls with ADHD. Already feeling misunderstood and fearful of rejection, the possibility of a *false self* that might help them gain acceptance is an attractive proposition. As a result, girls with ADHD are very likely to develop a protective façade as a way of compensating for their differences. It is a defense that may seem to offer an interpersonal buffer, but that façade comes at a high price. Whether the defense takes the form of compliance, arrogance, or aloofness, the outcome can be dire: their *true self* is never known, acknowledged, or validated. Over time, they begin to feel like impostors who dread discovery.

Unlike relationships with parents and teachers, peer interactions allow children to learn to cooperate and negotiate with parties of equal status. The development of these skills is critical for successful social functioning, and problematic peer relationships increase the risk for a wide variety of negative outcomes.[15] Despite equivalent executive functioning impairments and ADHD symptoms, inattention is related to poorer peer interactions for girls, but not for boys. In addition, ADHD patterns have more negative effects on peer acceptance for girls compared to boys. They have also been shown to experience much higher levels of peer victimization than boys with ADHD or girls without ADHD.[16] Whether they interrupt, are too blunt, messy at lunch, too competitive in sports, or miss subtle social cues, they are not demonstrating behaviors that have been deemed appropriately *feminine.* As a result of the differential cultural tolerance for these behaviors from girls versus boys, girls with ADHD are more likely to be rejected, clearly placing them at risk for continuing social problems.[17] Unfortunately, there is evidence that impaired social relationships have a more detrimental impact on the overall development of girls with ADHD compared to boys with ADHD, and that those difficulties persist into adolescence.[18]

INTERNALIZING SYMPTOMS

Following suit with the tendency of middle school girls to silence their own voices, many girls with ADHD begin to internalize their fears and disappointments, rather than talking it out or acting it out. In fact, girls with ADHD are more likely to experience coexisting internalizing symptoms than either boys with ADHD or girls without ADHD.[20, 21, 22] This tendency towards internalization serves to obscure most observable ADHD symptoms, especially in more inattentive girls. Instead, some of the more easily observed manifestations of internalized anxiety, rapid speech, irritability, restlessness, avoidant behavior, ruminating or obsessing, exaggerated fears, difficulty sleeping, episodes of panic, headaches and stomachaches emerge. Unaddressed, these tendencies can place them at significant risk of developing a discrete internalizing disorder in adolescence,[23] with inattentive girls more likely to develop Separation Anxiety Disorder.[24] The most common internalized symptoms related to low self-esteem are isolation and withdrawal, guilt and shame, and depressive feelings, including tearfulness and excessive sleeping.[25, 26] Repeated experience with underachievement and isolation can result in feelings of despair and demoralization.[27] When ADHD goes unaddressed, these girls can lose hope, and the more impulsive girls may act on those hopeless feelings.[28]

It has been shown that girls with ADHD, who exhibit internalizing symptoms, consistently received negative social ratings compared to boys exhibiting similar symptoms. Whether the raters were peers, teachers, or parents, it was the internalizing symptoms, rather than the ADHD symptoms themselves, that seemed to elicit the negative responses.[29] This suggests that internalizing symptoms may play a particularly important role in the trajectory of ADHD, especially for girls.

SELF-REPORT TOOLS NEEDED TO ASSESS INTERNALIZED SYMPTOMS

Internalized symptoms represent abstract experiences that are difficult to observe, recognize, describe, and label. In addition, girls with ADHD cannot know that the quality of their inner lives differs from that of other girls, and may assume that their anxious or depressive feelings are *normal.* For these reasons, they may not generate descriptions of internalized symptoms independently, but they can respond to prompts. To that end, a comprehensive assessment should evaluate internalizing (and externalizing) symptoms, in addition to ADHD symptoms. Whether a girl's internalized symptoms are secondary to ADHD, or have reached the level of a disorder, the nearly ubiquitous presence of internalizing conditions calls for self-assessments in addition to parent assessments.[30] These important experiences cannot be tapped by parent or teacher report, and highlight the value of our self-report questionnaires, which offer clinicians a necessary window into the inner lives of girls with ADHD.

EXTERNALIZING SYMPTOMS

For the more impulsive girls with ADHD, middle school is the time when externalizing symptoms become more noticeable. Although girls with ADHD exhibit less externalizing behaviors than boys with ADHD, parents and teachers report more difficulties with the oppositional behaviors of middle school girls with ADHD compared to those of boys with ADHD.[31] This may reflect the adults' lack of comfort with externalizing behaviors that are less gender typical for middle school age girls. The oppositional and/or aggressive behaviors exhibited by these girls tend to be more covert, such as lying, stealing, or verbal abuse, compared to boys' behaviors, which feature more overt physical aggression and rule-breaking.[32] These impulsive girls are more likely to be diagnosed with oppositional defiant disorder than girls without ADHD.[33, 34]

THE IMPACT OF PUBERTY

While the physiological effects of hormonal changes are discussed in Chapter Three, the psychological complexities of puberty pose another layer of challenges. For girls with ADHD, emotional maturity lags significantly behind physical maturity, leaving them psychologically unprepared to deal with their developing bodies. Just as they were developing workable coping strategies, hormonal changes create unpredictable emotional volatility for these girls.[35] Many deny their bodily changes, resisting the transition into unknown territory. Suddenly, they are barraged by novel and awkward situations, such as having to contend with bras, remembering to use deodorant, and towering over boys. Coping with the complexities of menstruation in school undermines almost all girls with ADHD at this age. In addition, impulse-driven sexual feelings are awakening and create tremendous internal confusion and distraction. Parents may find themselves in a worrisome situation as their very immature and impulsive daughters develop alluring curves and start showing interest in boys. Managing the heightened emotional and physiological sensitivities of puberty and integrating them into their developing sense of self makes this upheaval one of the defining challenges of the middle school years for girls with ADHD.

ACADEMIC CHALLENGES

In middle school, girls with ADHD are faced with abrupt changes to the familiar academic structures: a more complex curriculum, multiple teachers and classrooms, navigating crowded halls under strict time pressure, large backpacks, and locker combinations. These transitions are particularly difficult for girls with ADHD, and the emotional climate is less overtly nurturing, with less guidance and greater expectations of independent functioning. In and out of class, social interactions increase in complexity, fueled by hormonal awareness and emotional hyperreactivity. There are sudden demands for increased self-direction, greater organization, more efficient memory, appropriate prioritizing, and quicker transitions. It has been shown that the ability to rely on the executive functions is critical for managing these new levels of complexity, and it is the area where girls with ADHD are at a disadvantage.[36] Middle school girls with ADHD have been shown to have greater executive dysfunction than non-ADHD peers, regardless of subtype,[37] and those neuropsychological deficits persist into adolescence.[38]

The symptoms of inattention in middle school have been shown to strongly increase the risk for educational underachievement, regardless of the presence of hyperactivity.[39] In addition, executive dysfunction, which commonly co-occurs with ADHD, increases the risk for lower academic achievement, grade retention, and learning disabilities.[40] As a result, it is not surprising that the cognitive functioning of girls with ADHD is more impaired than that of girls without ADHD, as reflected in lower IQ, lower grade point average, lower motivation, and lower academic expectations.[41, 42] Compared to their peers, girls with ADHD exhibit poorer performance on measures of working memory, planning, and cognitive flexibility, although the pattern of deficits may change over time.[43] Although there are few neuropsychological gender differences in middle school students with ADHD, girls are at a higher risk of having speech and language disorders than boys,[44] with a significantly higher risk of written language disorders when accompanied by reading disabilities.[45] They also exhibit more difficulty with planning, including tasks without immediate teacher feedback,[46] and visual/spatial planning[47] than boys with ADHD.

WHAT TEACHERS SEE

The more inattentive girls with ADHD generally follow explicit rules and keep a low profile. Easily alienated and overwhelmed, their peers view them as being shy, and they experience more social isolation than their non-ADHD peers.[48] Avoiding class participation and eye contact, they hide in the back of the room, hoping that the teacher doesn't interrupt their daydreaming with a question they feel ill-prepared to answer. When frustrated with their work, they tend to surrender quickly, rather than ask for help, and they tend to be forgetful in terms of homework assignments. Their consequent underachievement reflects their lack of engagement with their studies, but it is easily misconstrued as a lack of ability.

Symptoms of inattentiveness are hallmarks of ADHD in girls, yet these more subtle symptoms elicit less attention from teachers than characteristically more disruptive ADHD symptoms seen in boys. In one study, teachers identified those with inattentive ADHD as the least impaired, and girls with hyperactive and impulsive symptoms as the most impaired compared to boys with ADHD.[49] This may be, in part, because girls' inattentive symptoms are not recognized as typical indications of ADHD and partly because these symptoms are less noticeable and troublesome to teachers than are boys' symptoms. Combined with the tendency of these girls to suffer silently and not ask for help, their fate may be that they are less likely to be referred for evaluation, and that they may bear the burden of untreated ADHD for a much longer time than do boys.

Indeed, in a national survey of 550 teachers, almost half said that it is harder for them to recognize ADHD symptoms in girls than in boys. The teachers reported that most schools (90%) provided little or no training on ADHD.[50] In fact, teachers reported more difficulties with oppositional behavior, conduct problems, social difficulties, anxiety, and depression in girls with ADHD compared to boys with ADHD. In other words, the teachers were responding to the psychological impairments that can coexist with ADHD, rather than to core ADHD symptoms themselves. They identified physiological internalizing symptoms such as anxiety as the most important non-ADHD symptom that helped them distinguish girls with ADHD from non-ADHD girls.[51]

In middle school, overt hyperactivity gives way to more subtle physical manifestations like fine-motor fidgeting, hair twirling, cuticle picking, nail biting, and frequent doodling. Many girls can stay seated but experience an uncomfortable sense of internal restlessness, leading them to constantly check the clock. These more impulsive girls with ADHD are more prone to rule-breaking, feeling confined and limited by the rules rather than structured and supported by them. More oppositional and aggressive than the inattentive girls, the impulsive girls may come to identify themselves as belonging amongst those who violate social norms. They may discover that they can find acceptance with peers who also violate societal norms. Instead of fighting their impulses, they connect via a shared activity, as well as by their willingness to engage in high-risk behaviors that involve rebellious rule violations. It makes sense, then, that the more impulsive middle school girls with ADHD are often among the first to experiment with cigarettes, alcohol, drugs, or sex as avenues to peer acceptance. Alarmingly, for some, these patterns can begin as early as age eleven, although most begin these explorations in middle school.[52]

GIRLS WITH A HIGH IQ

While a frequent topic of controversy, it has been shown that high IQ children can also meet the diagnostic criteria for ADHD.[53, 54] Very bright girls with ADHD were probably able to coast through elementary school, compensating for their ADHD symptoms with relatively little effort. The teaching style in the elementary grades emphasizes highly structured lessons utilizing visual materials as well as hands-on experiences, which play to the strengths of most girls with ADHD. While they may have felt awkward inside, academic challenges were probably not experienced as particularly demanding and their achievement was likely to be impressive. Their school performance was likely a reliable source of self-esteem, even if the social realm was less rewarding.

It is most often during middle school that these high IQ girls begin to falter. Brown and colleagues have shown that high IQ children with ADHD also suffer from executive dysfunction, and have significant weaknesses in working memory and processing speed. Nonetheless, their high IQ allows them to compensate for these difficulties, resulting in later diagnosis and treatment.[55] Regardless of their innate intelligence or acquired knowledge, the very smart girls with ADHD still require more time, practice, and effort than their peers to consistently manage these demands.

These smart girls had previously defined themselves in terms of their superior intellects and gathered some self-esteem from that status. Now they see less gifted peers better able to achieve while they struggle. They can't understand why they suddenly have to work so hard without attaining the expected successes. Some cling self-righteously to rules; when they witness impulsive rule-breakers, they can be quite harsh and rigid in their judgments. They tend to feel shame about their changing status. Underachievement can become a self-perpetuating theme that often continues throughout adolescence, creating confusion and undermining self-esteem. No longer identifying with the smart kids, they need to find a new way to fit in with their peers.

THE MINEFIELD OF SOCIAL LIFE

The desire to be accepted by peers is particularly intense for middle school girls; however, girls with poor executive functioning have a high risk of poor social functioning.[56] Middle school girls with ADHD experience more social impairment and peer victimization than girls without ADHD.[57,58] They are more likely to have problems with conduct, mood, anxiety, and language than girls without ADHD, all of which can have a negative impact on peer relationships.[59] They are more likely to be verbally aggressive toward their peers than either boys with ADHD[61] or non-ADHD girls.[62] In addition, they are more likely to engage in relational aggression than girls without ADHD.[63,64] Compared to inattentive boys with ADHD, inattentive girls are at a higher risk for being bullied; they tend to be less popular and have worse peer relationships.[65] Although ADHD symptoms and executive dysfunction clearly contribute to the development of girls' social problems, it seems that they do not fully account for the social impairments they experience.[66]

RELATIONAL AGGRESSION

Relational aggression occurs when the relationship is used as the vehicle of harm. For middle school girls, common scenarios involve spreading malicious gossip, compelling others not to talk to someone, telling someone they cannot join your group, or using ultimatums like "I won't be your friend unless you..." These covert attacks on friendship capitalize on the monumental importance of intimacy exchange for girls, rendering it a particularly effective means of manipulating middle school girls.[67] Even in a computerized social interaction game that removes the intensity of direct communication, girls with ADHD were more overtly aggressive, relationally aggressive and socially awkward than comparison girls.[68]

As most girls acquire increasingly more sophisticated social and cognitive skills toward the end of elementary school, they are able to engage in more intimate relationships with friends. Girls with ADHD are delayed in developing these abilities, so they are just beginning to explore closer friendships in middle school. Unfortunately, this more intimate knowledge of their friends provides them with ammunition that is used against their friends. Indeed, it has been shown that girls use relational aggression against their close friends; high levels of intimacy and exclusivity within a friendship actually increase the likelihood of relational aggression.[69]

One study found that girls with at least one friend were less likely to experience peer victimization, defined as frequent verbal or relational harassment of weaker age-mates. This was true for girls with or without ADHD, and their risk of victimization was reduced whether or not the friend had ADHD.[70] A further study demonstrated that the risk of social problems was lower when the girls perceived that their best friendship included high rates of disclosure and emotional support. In other words, the quality of the friendship was protective, rather than the existence of the relationship itself. Specifically, the sense of having a true intimacy exchange made the friendship of a higher quality, which lowered the risk of social problems for girls with ADHD.[71]

Unfortunately, protection from peer victimization does not reduce the negative effects of peer rejection. In fact, early peer rejection increases the risk for delinquency, depression, anxiety, substance use, and general impairment by middle school.[72] For middle school girls with ADHD, relational aggression is related to internalizing symptoms, whether they are the perpetrator or the target.[73] Studies suggest that peer rejection increases the risk for future psychological problems in adolescence, such as eating disorders.[74] Nonetheless, girls with ADHD desperately crave friendship and a sense of belonging. Fueled by these motivations, they are willing to go to great lengths to make themselves attractive to others. They may make poignant attempts by offering jewelry to the popular girls, or by joining a dance class in which they have no interest or ability, just to be in the orbit of the desirable girls. When they perceive that they are unable to conform to the social expectations of their peers, they begin to seek other routes to connection.

THE POWER OF SEXUALITY

By this age, many girls with ADHD are resigned to being unpopular; at best, they cling to the fringes of social groups and, at worst, they are routinely rejected and bullied. Just when the situation appears hopeless, they discover that boys who never acknowledged them before are suddenly friendly and attentive. Due to the lags in social and emotional development, they initially see this male interest as platonic, and respond enthusiastically. Many middle school girls with ADHD say, "I don't know why, but all of my best friends are boys," and they may even enjoy being accepted as one of the boys. For girls who have never enjoyed social successes where they have been sought out and made to feel special, this is a tremendously powerful experience. This can be a dizzying combination of overwhelming feelings and impulses — all of it providing very high stimulation.

Soon, they may proudly state that they have a boyfriend, without an understanding of that commitment. If they are lucky, they will have the chance to gradually understand the sexual urges that accompany male puberty. Many girls with ADHD decide that the benefits of early sexual experimentation have worthwhile payoffs. Some find the intensity of these interactions difficult to resist, and may become promiscuous. Videos, music lyrics, and young teen celebrities all reinforce the triumph in these sexual goals. Unfortunately, girls with ADHD can easily get in over their heads, and parents should be vigilant about providing oversight during parties, private online chats, and text messaging. The combination of high stimulation, hormonal changes, and social rewards can lead to an addictive involvement in sexual acting out.

THE LOVE/HATE RELATIONSHIP WITH FOOD

Like their sexuality, managing food consumption involves impulse regulation that girls with ADHD wrestle with on a daily basis. Preoccupation with weight concerns, body dissatisfaction, and interest in dieting reflects adherence to today's gender role ideals[75] as they pursue society's unforgiving model of female attractiveness.[76] They tend to judge themselves harshly as they compare themselves to others, and experience guilt, shame, anxiety, and low self-esteem. Shari's story is typical of a middle school girl with ADHD.

Shari, an eighth grader, still hadn't received an invitation to Rebecca's party. It was already Thursday and the party was Saturday; could she still get an invitation this late? She wasn't invited; she knew it, but didn't want to face it. She had listened attentively when the girls at school talked about what they were going to wear to the party, and she had smiled knowingly. And she knew that David would be there.

Now, she stared at herself in the mirror, and decided they didn't invite her because she was too fat. She was just turning to see her rear view when her brother, Matt, flung the door open without knocking. Shari screamed, "Get out, or I'll kill you!" Matt ran out, slamming the door behind him. From the impact, the plaster flower she had painted at Karen's birthday party crashed to the floor and broke. Shari looked down and burst into tears. When she heard Matt leave the house, she quietly went down to the kitchen. She searched the refrigerator frantically but nothing appealed to her. Then, she looked in the pantry and saw the chocolate chip cookies. Her mom had said that the cookies were for dessert tonight, when Uncle Phil came over. Shari decided she could have a few cookies and there'd be plenty left. She didn't want anyone to see her eating them, so she took them back up to her room. She turned up the music on her computer and ate the first cookie in two bites. She did the same thing with the next five. Soon, she started to feel calmer, and she forgot about Uncle Phil, and Mom, and Matt. She forgot that she had been dieting for two weeks for Rebecca's party. When all the cookies were gone, she began to rationalize why she didn't want to go to the party anyway. Not realizing that it was the day before her period, she convinced her-

self that she never really liked Rebecca anyway. It was a full five minutes before she started to feel guilty. Later, when her mom asked her if she had seen the cookies, she said "No" and quickly walked upstairs to her room. She looked at herself in the mirror as she walked in, and got upset all over again.

SOCIAL DILEMMAS ONLINE

For girls with ADHD who are daunted by the social complexities of middle school, online social networking offers opportunities to try out different personas. Online gaming is another avenue that allows admission into a socially acceptable subculture that enables even those with the poorest social skills to participate. The internet provides so much, that middle school girls can spend hours daily engaged in their online passions. Many parents question whether their daughters actually have ADHD because they can sustain attention to the internet over long periods of time. That ability becomes possible when the executive functions are able to work together in response to a stimulating combination of factors: constantly changing multisensory stimuli, immediate and varied rewards, and easy exit when overwhelmed, irritated, or bored. For these reasons, these girls can be thoroughly engaged online but can barely maintain focus long enough to get through their homework.

Middle school girls with ADHD may perceive that the internet promises experiences with social acceptance, all from the safety of their rooms. However, it has been shown that girls utilize the internet and texting to bully other girls and those girls with ADHD who are targets of traditional bullying experience the same problems online. In fact, girls with ADHD who are the targets of electronic victimization are almost always targeted in traditional ways as well, and this victimization contributes to the development of depression.[77]

Middle school girls with ADHD who are curious about sexuality can find what may seem to be similarly searching peer groups on the internet. It may feel more comfortable to them than trying to broach the topic with their peers. Essentially, unsupervised sites are easily available, with countless distorted facts and misinformation. The highly sexualized chats are a source of curiosity and arousal for these girls. Unfortunately, there are many pitfalls to this approach; they may feel pressured by those on the site to respond in ways that are outside of their comfort zone. They may impulsively offer personal information, up the ante of sexual challenges, miss important social cues, and fail to consider the possibility of predators. In fact, for girls, ADHD has been shown to increase the likelihood of internet addiction more than any other factor. Whether it is social networking, gaming, or sexualized chat rooms, it is the obsessive preoccupation and monumental time investment that can undermine healthy functioning.[78]

DESPERATE FOR ACCEPTANCE

While middle school girls with ADHD are not actively seeking out a problematic subculture, it becomes a worthwhile trade-off for them if they finally gain acceptance into a peer group. Even the girls who are most tuned out and withdrawn can be drawn into the excitement and rewards of this secret life. Each of these groups has its own subculture, its own jargon, its own societal rules—it's like a club for members only, and their acceptance as a member makes these girls feel special. These activities demand large time commitments and, for girls with ADHD who already struggle with time management, academics will begin to suffer. Even the daily risks of avoiding detection can be experienced as high stimulation by the ADHD brain. In fact, navigating these risks can even provide a sense of efficacy as well as social success. A full discussion of addictive behaviors that may coexist with ADHD can be found in Chapter Thirteen.

HOW TO INTERVENE

Armed with stimulating behaviors that open the doors to peer acceptance, girls with ADHD may even flaunt their involvement. Sadly, due to their impulsivity, this poor judgment can result in middle school girls with ADHD being the ones caught before other children in their group, or labeled negatively by their peers. When these behaviors ultimately come to light, it is helpful for parents to remember that the most compelling attraction for their daughters was initially the social group. Parents understandably focus on the risks of their daughters becoming more deeply involved with dangerous behaviors. However, intervention won't be effective unless it addresses the loss of the social connections as well. For the complex needs of girls with ADHD, breaking addictions is painful, but so is severing connections to a lifestyle that offered them acceptance.

A way to offer an alternative ADHD-friendly environment is to help them get involved in structured and supervised activities. Whether it is a sports activity, a community service organization, a religious youth group, or a drama group, these activities provide a built-in peer group. Adults circumscribe the activity, the time frame, and the ground rules for interactions. Usually, the inattentive types prefer activities that occur in a small intimate group; the more hyperemotional types can play to a larger and more varied audience. And, in the event that there is the inevitable misunderstanding with a peer, there will be a good number of potential acquaintances that remain. An activity imposes another piece of routine on her life and offers another arena for gaining self-esteem. This is especially valuable if her school performance is flagging and doesn't provide a source of pride at this time. Finally, from a practical standpoint, involvement in sanctioned activities will offer her less time and incentive to pursue riskier avenues. Parents can reinforce the importance of these activities by showing their support, whether by participating in a carpool to get her there, being present at the team games, or volunteering to supervise or chaperone, just to name a few possibilities.

It's easy for parents to miss the early signs that their daughters may be moving towards a problematic peer group. Parents may be focused on the decline in academic performance and not see it as symptomatic of a bigger picture. Parents who smoke or drink may not initially consider these behaviors as signs of danger. Parents may be in denial because they perceive their daughters as too young or innocent to be involved in undesirable activities. However, there are things that parents can do to increase their own awareness. First and foremost, be aware of changes in your daughters' social interactions. Do they suddenly have a new friend? They may change their *look* in some way — clothing, hair, makeup, tattoos, etc., or refuse to wear things that had been favorites. They may become more secretive about the ways they spend their free time, or about where they are during those hours. There are many films that treat the issues of middle school social struggles with sensitivity. Watching a film like *Mean Girls* with your daughter can open up a more general avenue for communication.

ADHD COACHES

A coach can be a helpful addition to the support network for middle school girls with ADHD. When parents are in the position of being the police who must enforce rules around responsibilities, it interferes with the emotional safety and joyfulness of the relationship with their daughters. If an ADHD coach is following up on the girl's responsibilities, parents are freer to remove themselves from the intense power struggle that is inevitable. While negotiating is a necessity, the role of policeman is better left to someone who does not share the emotional investment in your daughters' success. An all too familiar scenario was described by Terry's father.

> *"When I get home in the evening, I'm in charge of the homework detail. Terry argues about everything, whether or not she has homework, how much homework she has, how long it will take her to do it, what time she should start it, when she should take a break. You can't imagine the battles we have. After I haven't seen her all day, I hate for this to be the basis of our relationship, and often we are struggling up until her bedtime. We both agree that I have become more of a policeman than a dad, and neither of us likes it. I was complaining about this to Terry's psychologist and she suggested we try a coach. Since we hired Julie, my interactions with Terry are fun and loving, and she gets her work done too. A coach is one of the best investments I've ever made."*

As discussed, this is the age when girls begin to lose their voice. Parents can reinforce the value of that inner voice, and support the strength that is needed to maintain it amidst a culture that tends to silence girls. As mentioned earlier, research shows that levels of anxiety and depression increase at the end of middle school for girls with ADHD.[79] As these girls make the transition into adolescence, they struggle to plant their feet firmly beneath them. Whether they lurch in all directions at once, or pull back into a turtle shell, no one can protect them from being buffeted about by unpredictable winds. Ultimately, girls with ADHD must learn for themselves that they cannot change the wind, but they can learn to adjust their sails.

THE MESSAGES THAT MATTER MOST

While peer approval is paramount for this age group, the intensity of that need can be modulated. Work toward making your home a safe and available haven where your daughter will feel comfortable enough to discuss her concerns. If girls have a solid mother-daughter relationship in which they feel accepted and supported, they are less likely to allow peers alone to define their self-worth. Certainly, the mother's tightrope act of supporting her daughter's separation and growing independence on the one hand, and the desire to protect her daughter from pain, on the other hand, is one of the most bittersweet passages of parenthood. Speaking frankly with her about the changes in her body and her feelings lets her know that these things are normal; and not one more thing that makes her different. Acknowledging that middle school is a confusing time, with lots of new feelings and distractions, will validate her experience.

Expect comments like "It's not fair," and "You just don't understand." Expect frequent withdrawal from the family, with your daughter closeted in her room. Expect rolling of the eyes as the default response to almost any parental statement, and frustration, sarcasm, and irritability to anything resembling parental control. Because they tend to conceptualize the world into black and white dichotomies, expect that compromise will not seem an acceptable option. Now, with increasing hormones comes increasing intensity and increasing reactivity. One mother described her daughter Pam in this way: "She starts to cry over something that seems so minor, and soon it turns into hysterical sobbing. Later, she says, 'You know, you can't treat me like a kid anymore.'" Teetering on the boundary between childhood and young womanhood, her body tells her she is no longer a kid, but her behavior often betrays her.

Mothers can normalize their daughters' experiences by letting them know that even you felt the same way when you were their age. Above all, give the consistent message that you accept them as they are and will support them. This doesn't mean that you approve of their behaviors. There may well be behaviors that concern you, confuse you, or scare you, and that you should discuss with her father, other family, friends, and professionals. Brief family counseling is often useful to get some ground rules in place. But the message to your daughters must be that you do not judge them or reject them, as so much of their world does. In order to nurture this relationship of trust, your message needs to be consistent — if they believe that you embrace them as they are, they will reveal their vulnerabilities to you.

QUESTIONS TO ASK YOURSELF ABOUT YOUR MIDDLE SCHOOL DAUGHTER

This list is designed to aid parents who may wonder about the possibility of ADHD in their middle school daughters. We ask you to consider your daughter with these questions in mind. Even if you answer "Yes" to many of the following questions, it does not necessarily indicate that your daughter has ADHD. However, if your concern is aroused, it may be advisable to seek the advice of a professional.

- Does she daydream frequently?
- Does she have trouble getting started on her homework?
- Is she easily distracted from mundane activities?
- Does she forget things she's supposed to do?
- Does she seem resistant to reading for pleasure?
- Does she seem oversensitive and easily embarrassed?
- Is she generally disorganized?
- Is it a struggle to get her up in the morning?
- Does she often have a physical complaint, such as a headache or stomachache?
- Is she often late for school or other activities?
- Does she march to the beat of a different drummer?
- Does she usually stay up later at night than you'd like?
- Does she often lose or misplace items?
- Does she stay at the fringe of a large group activity?
- Does she wish she had more friends?
- Does she often lose track of the time?
- Does she tend to be shy with her peers?
- Does she seem forgetful or absent-minded?

- Does she leave a trail of belongings throughout the house?
- Does she have a low frustration tolerance?
- Does she tend to interrupt conversations?
- Does she seem immature for her age?
- Does her teacher say she should speak up in class or try harder?
- Does she quickly become annoyed or irritable?
- Does she seem to overreact?
- Does she tend to put things off until later?
- Does she often seem like she's not listening when you speak to her?
- Does she tend to blame others rather than accept responsibility?
- Is she thrown off by transitions?

CHAPTER SIX

The High School Years
More Demands and Greater Risks for Girls with ADHD

AS HAS BEEN SHOWN FOR BOYS,[1-3] most girls diagnosed with ADHD during the elementary school years do not grow out of it by adolescence.[4,5] As a result, the high school years can be a difficult and challenging time for adolescents with ADHD.[6] It seems as if nature and society have conspired to pack these four years with so many daunting challenges that even the most adept and well-adjusted adolescent feels overloaded. When ADHD is added to the mix, high school becomes more challenging, and may even turn out to be a negative experience for the adolescent with ADHD.

In this chapter, we examine the particular vulnerabilities for girls with ADHD in high school and suggest ways that parents, teachers, and other professionals can offer much-needed support.

ADJUSTMENT IN ADOLESCENCE FOR GIRLS DIAGNOSED WITH ADHD

Girls diagnosed with ADHD during their early years are substantially less likely to be well-adjusted during adolescence.[7] To estimate the prevalence of being well-adjusted in adolescence, boys and girls with and without ADHD were assessed seven times in eight years starting when they were four to six years of age. Symptoms of ADHD, ODD/CD, and depression/anxiety in addition to social skills and social preference were gathered using multiple methods and informants. Being well-adjusted was defined by surpassing thresholds in at least four of the five domains. At the seven- and eight-year follow-ups, when youth were 11-14 years old, those with ADHD were significantly less likely to be well-adjusted relative to age- and ethnicity-matched control children. Only a minority of children with ADHD were well-adjusted in adolescence when emotional, behavioral, and social domains were considered simultaneously. Even when their ADHD symptoms improved over time, most children with ADHD exhibited significant impairment in adolescence, seven to eight years after their initial assessment.

In a study published in 2009, when girls with ADHD were compared to girls without ADHD, the majority of those with ADHD were found to be poorly adjusted. Researchers measured adjustment in girls with and without ADHD in multiple domains — ADHD symptoms, behavior problems, internalizing problems (i.e., depressive and anxiety symptoms), social skills, peer relationships, and academic functioning, and defined overall positive adjustment (PA) when girls showed average scores in five of these domains. Using these criteria, only 16% of girls with the ADHD were found to have overall PA in adolescence compared to 86% of non-ADHD girls.[8]

Researchers also considered whether the type of ADHD (inattentive vs. combined) made any difference in adjustment. Interestingly, girls with the inattentive type tended to be less likely to show overall PA in adolescence at this five-year follow-up compared to combined type girls. They also examined the association between being in treatment in the past year and overall PA in girls with ADHD. Predictably, girls with ADHD that were doing less well in terms of PA were more likely to be in treatment, taking medication and/or receiving psychotherapy.[9] Overall, these results speak to the chronic nature of the symptoms and impairments associated with childhood ADHD for girls. However, it's important for parents to remember that a sizable minority of the girls in these studies were doing well despite their ADHD and rated in the positively adjusted group. It is, therefore, important to remember that although a childhood diagnosis of ADHD often predicts continuing difficulty, such outcomes are by no means inevitable. Let's take a look at some of the reasons girls with ADHD may be having difficulties with adjustment in these various domains during adolescence.

HIGH SCHOOL AND ADHD NOT A GOOD FIT

Pressures and academic demands seem to reach a crescendo in high school because there is so little choice and flexibility. High school is designed in a way that seems almost diabolically structured to be ADHD-unfriendly. The day starts too early and lasts too long — with demands for focus, concentration, and organization that far exceed the capacity of most students, even those without ADHD. There is little choice in the array of courses required for graduation. Many students with ADHD are placed in the position of being forced to read about and study subjects that hold little or no interest for them — something they should be strongly advised against doing once they have graduated from high school! And yet, during the high school years, they don't have many options to customize their courses and activities. As a result, adolescents with ADHD display numerous academic problems.

According to parent and teacher reports, adolescents with ADHD displayed problematic academic behaviors in multiple daily tasks, with time management and planning deficits appearing most pervasive.[10] Academic performance is most likely affected by continued executive functioning (EF) deficits. In follow-up studies of girls diagnosed in childhood, deficits in executive functioning (including planning, organization, inhibitory control, sustained attention, working memory, and set shifting) were found to continue through adolescence [11] and into young adulthood.[12] At the later follow-up, EF deficits were found to be independent of type of ADHD presentation (combined vs. inattentive) or in those girls whose symptoms of ADHD persisted versus those whose symptoms had remitted and who no longer received the diagnosis of ADHD.

INCREASING SOCIAL PRESSURES IN ADOLESCENCE

Social deficits, seen during earlier years, often have their greatest impact during adolescence as girls begin to separate from family and move into the all-important social milieu of high school. During the high school years, girls begin to move out of the all-girl cliques of middle school and begin to explore their individuality in both same sex and opposite sex relationships. The more complex high school social patterns often call for a level of awareness and self-control that many girls with ADHD don't possess. Their social deficits result in the sad, but common tale told by women with ADHD — that they were never quite able to navigate successfully in their high school social sphere.

Social pressures are intense for all students during adolescence, with enormous energy expended on peer analysis: watching, imitating, relating, comparing, and conforming. In addition to this exhausting process, girls with ADHD often feel despair. Recalling their adolescent years, the phrases we hear repeated again and again by women with ADHD are, "I didn't fit in," or, "I always felt different, but I never knew why." Many report having "no friends" or only "one best friend," while others recall their adolescent years as a blur of impulsive behavior, promiscuity, and heavy drinking in a desperate effort to gain acceptance. Those who did manage to succeed academically often had no time at all for social life, paying an extra high price for top grades.

> *"In high school I was shy and really didn't have any friends. I just felt like I never fit in with any type of people. I didn't feel I was smart, but I never wanted to hang out with the 'rough crowd' either."*

Family support and acceptance is critical, but can never entirely counteract the damage that can be done to teenagers who feel rejected by their peer group. The very negative self-image that girls with ADHD may develop during high school can haunt them for years afterwards. This pattern presents a strong argument for providing group treatment for adolescent girls with ADHD. Such a social setting can provide what is likely the first peer group that offers understanding and acceptance, in addition to being a safe place to learn coping skills and strategies to reduce ADHD challenges.

This treatment suggestion is supported by the results from a recent study conducted to evaluate the social behavior of adolescents with ADHD in single and mixed gender treatment settings.[13] Ratings of social behavior (i.e., prosocial peer interactions, assertiveness, self-management, compliance, physical aggression, relational aggression) were collected during single and mixed gender games within a summer treatment program for adolescents. Counselors completed ratings immediately following 10 recreational periods for each adolescent they supervised. Several very interesting interactions emerged, suggesting that girls benefited more from single rather than mixed gender formats. Girls showed more assertiveness, self-management, and compliance in single gender formats.

GENDER EXPECTATIONS ARE OFTEN IN DIRECT CONFLICT WITH ADHD TRAITS

If we examine some of the pressures and expectations often placed on teenage girls, it is easy to see how they can come into direct conflict with ADHD traits or tendencies. For example, girls are typically encouraged to be neat, feminine (controlled and passive), carefully groomed (in order to be attractive to the opposite sex), sensitive to the feelings of others, and compliant toward adults. In his book, *The Triple Bind*, Dr. Steven Hinshaw discusses the crisis faced by teenaged girls as a result of the expectations placed on them today. First, they must "be good at all the traditional girl stuff ...relationships ...empathy...and bonding." Second, they must "be good at most of the traditional guy stuff ...fighting for spots at top colleges, preparing themselves for the job market, and playing at sports." Third, they must conform to a narrow, unrealistic set of standards that allows for no alternative." Given the triple threat, he postulated that it's no wonder that today's girls are at risk, with 25% at immediate danger for eating disorders, self-injury, depression, and suicide.[14]

As a result of these pressures, a teenage girl with ADHD may respond anxiously, even obsessively, to these expectations. She may be unable to organize her room or her life well enough to have clean, color-coordinated clothing available on a given school morning. This may lead to frantic, screaming tirades as she searches through piles of clothing on the floor, the dirty clothesbasket, or her sister's closet. She may impulsively grab something to wear at the last minute, as she races out the door for school—very likely leaving behind some crucial item in her rush.

The self-doubts and competitiveness, so common among teenage girls, are often more intense for girls with ADHD. Hurt feelings can escalate more rapidly into impulsive remarks or over-reactions. Studies have shown that girls with ADHD may be verbally aggressive rather than physically aggressive like males with ADHD.[15] However, once the drama is over, a girl with ADHD may be ready to forgive and forget. Yet she often finds herself facing rejection by peers who having been stung by her comments are no longer tolerant of her outbursts.

Of course, there is overlap between the dilemmas of teenage boys and girls with ADHD. Girls aren't the only ones who may feel socially excluded. But girls seem to feel much more intense reactions to social difficulties than do boys with ADHD during adolescence. This may, in part, be due to the fact that ADHD-like behaviors, such as risk-taking, arguing, defiance, and being action-oriented, are more socially acceptable for boys. Similar traits in girls, however, can be met with criticism, and even ostracism.

Boys may engage in group activities or group sports without being required to exhibit the same level of social skills that are expected from a girl. Patterns of interrupting, contradicting, or reacting angrily rarely result in social ostracism among boys, unless these behaviors occur repeatedly or in the extreme. In addition, boys can often retreat behind athletics, or even behind a "Who cares?" attitude if social skills are lacking.

The goal in helping girls with ADHD during adolescence is for them to learn to value themselves, and to seek the company of people who can appreciate their strengths. Through building awareness of their strengths and special gifts, they can avoid falling into a pattern of self-reproach for their inability to measure up to the standards of social convention.

Parents and other professionals can provide much-needed support to adolescent girls with ADHD by engaging in social engineering — actively helping girls with ADHD to find safe social pockets within the overwhelming anxiety and competition of the high school social milieu. For example, one very bright, shy, inattentive-type girl found great solace in joining the local "It's Academic" team at her high school. These "brainiacs" lunched together daily, grilling each other in preparation for weekend competitions with other high school teams. Before joining this group, she avoided eating lunch altogether because entering the cafeteria having no friend to sit with created overwhelming anxiety. Another girl, with the support of her parents, completely embraced the world of horseback riding. She worked at the local stable grooming horses and mucking out stalls and found herself quite at home among the tomboyish, less appearance conscious girls that hung out at the barn. Yet another girl found that participation in the high school drama group gave her an outlet for her big voice, intense feelings, and oversized personality.

PRESSURES TO MATURE

Pressure to grow up and become responsible increases during adolescence. Sometimes parental expectations for their daughters to demonstrate maturity can come into direct conflict with the neurocognitive patterns associated with ADHD. This doesn't mean that our daughters can't become mature, but it does mean that maturity needs to be viewed through an ADHD lens. In other words, it is important to recognize those areas that pose a much greater challenge for girls with ADHD. What we call maturity typically involves the ability to make and follow plans, to postpone immediate gratification, to consider consequences, to moderate emotional reactions, to reliably do what we've been asked to do, to learn from the past, and to plan for the future. Many of these signs of maturity are capacities related to the executive functions of the frontal lobes of the brain, and it is the frontal lobes that are primarily affected by ADHD as discussed in Chapter Ten on Executive Functions and ADHD.

What does this mean to the adolescent girl with ADHD? She may be more forgetful, less reliable, and have much more difficulty in planning and carrying out long-term assignments. In general, she may be more prone to feel overwhelmed by the multiple demands of high school, extracurricular activities, social life, and part-time work. The hopeful news, however, is that frontal lobes continue to develop throughout adolescence and young adulthood, increasing her ability to effectively take charge of her life.

EXPECTATIONS FOR CONFORMITY AND COMPLIANCE

Many forces are at work for both boys and girls with ADHD, making it difficult for them to excel in high school. However, there is added pressure for girls because of their greater needs for social acceptance, for meeting the expectations of parents and teachers, as well as their overall greater desire to conform. Girls with ADHD may be more prone to anxiety—an outgrowth of this desire to please, to do what is expected. Their efforts to compensate in order to meet expectations may mask their ADHD struggles, making their difficulties more likely to be overlooked by parents and teachers. As it becomes increasingly challenging for girls with ADHD to meet expected demands, their anxiety levels often rise, and it becomes much more difficult for a girl to live with the consequences of ADHD and still feel good about herself.

All of the social conditioning that told her as a little girl that she should be good (sweet, compliant, clean, and tidy) doesn't disappear, even though it may seem so. If you are a parent who has daily screaming battles with your daughter, you may read this with skepticism. What great desire to conform? All she does is argue! Although she may be very emotionally volatile and may strongly resist your attempts to control her, she still lives with an inner struggle. Your little girl, who had stomach aches because she couldn't manage to do what the teacher asked, is still alive and well somewhere inside. We know this through listening to the recollections of grown women with ADHD. Whether or not she lets you know it, it is likely that she feels deeply wounded when she is criticized by parents, teachers, and others. She may compare herself unfavorably to the successes of her peers, as well. Although as a teen she may feign indifference to negative opinions, later she will have painful recollections of this period of her life.

INCREASING EMOTIONAL REACTIVITY

Teenage girls with ADHD tend to be more emotionally reactive than other girls, and to have a harder time moderating the intensity of their responses. Whether it is frustration over a homework assignment, distress over her appearance, anger at a younger sibling who borrowed her sweater, despair over feeling socially isolated, or anger at parents who treat her like a baby, the emotional roller coaster that is adolescence tends to be more extreme for a girl with ADHD. Huessy, an early ADHD expert, writes that behavioral problems for many girls with ADHD only begin after puberty, accompanied by an increase in emotional over-reactivity, mood swings, and impulsivity.[16]

Hormonal changes occurring at puberty affect emotional volatility, leading many girls with ADHD to become emotionally hyperreactive. It is critical that parents and professionals recognize that this reactivity has a neurological basis, and that reactions tend to become even more extreme during times of stress, fatigue, hunger, or premenstrually, when hormones are undergoing change. Both the teenage girl and her parents need to recognize the added vulnerability that she has, and begin to identify and manage the potential stresses that can worsen her reactions.

THE IMPACT OF HORMONAL CHANGES

In a short, four-year period, our daughters with ADHD move from girlhood to the brink of womanhood. Tremendous hormonal changes occur, and the hormonal fluctuations of the menstrual cycle intensify and complicate the confusion and unpredictability that are part and parcel of growing up with ADHD. While premenstrual syndrome may be an annoying period of irritability, fatigue, or cramping for many girls, those with ADHD may feel such an increase in the intensity of their emotional reactions, irritability, and low frustration tolerance, that they require active intervention. Physicians, therapists and others who treat adolescent girls with ADHD should be aware of this added vulnerability, and take steps to keep up-to-date on research on PMS and on new approaches for minimizing its impact.

ADHD AS A LATER DIAGNOSIS IN GIRLS

While it is becoming more common for girls to be diagnosed in elementary school, many girls, particularly those who are very bright or who are growing up in a very supportive environment, often are not diagnosed until high school or later. Parents and professionals alike need to be aware of the reasons why a girl's symptoms may not be seen until age 12 and why a girl may not be diagnosed with ADHD until functioning is impaired when she begins to experience academic difficulties in high school or even college. The fact that ADHD symptoms may not have been apparent during her early years does not mean they were not present or render her ADHD diagnosis any less real. As a result, changes in DSM-5[17] reflect this later onset of the disorder. Girls with ADHD often behave very differently than boys with the disorder. Females may work harder to hide their academic difficulties and to conform to teacher expectations or develop coping strategies.[18] In such cases, symptoms of ADHD may not be seen until adolescence; a time when the demands for planning, organization, recall, and focus (executive functions) intensify.

As has been seen all too often, these girls become anxious or depressed as their ADHD symptoms impact their lives. Girls with ADHD are far more likely than non-diagnosed peers to maintain or develop internalizing and/or externalizing disorders in adolescence.[19-22] Self-esteem suffers and a whole host of other behaviors follow. As a result of these other behaviors, girls with ADHD are often misdiagnosed as anxious and/or depressed in adolescence, and subsequently treated for these disorders, while the real reason for their suffering, their ADHD, is missed. In one survey, 14% of girls with ADHD reported having taken antidepressants prior to their ADHD diagnosis compared with only 5% of boys.[23]

Unfortunately, skepticism is common on the part of educators even when a late diagnosis occurs. Girls who are diagnosed late may need extra support and advocacy from parents and professionals as they may encounter resistance when they request accommodations on standardized testing for college entrance, or as they need other accommodations and support during their high school years.

RISKS ASSOCIATED WITH ADHD IN ADOLESCENT GIRLS

As discussed earlier, Dr. Hinshaw has pointed out in his book, *The Triple Bind*, that adolescent girls today are in danger from self-injury, eating disorders, violence, depression, and suicide.[24]

Girls with ADHD are at an even greater risk for these and other conditions during later adolescence. ADHD with its symptoms of impulsivity, distractibility, poor decision-making, and difficulty planning ahead may lead to significant challenges for girls with ADHD during adolescence. Let's take a look at some of these risks and what parents can do to address or minimize them.

ADHD AND CONDUCT DISORDERS (CD) IN GIRLS

ADHD has been shown to be a significant risk factor for developing CD throughout childhood and adolescence.[25] In one study, childhood-onset CD was predicted by paternal antisocial personality disorder (ASPD), while adolescent-onset CD was predicted by family conflict. In addition, ADHD and CD in girls were associated with an increased risk for academic, psychiatric, and sexual behavior problems compared to ADHD girls without CD.[26] Given that the treatment approaches for ADHD and CD differ, these findings highlight the importance of improved efforts aimed at early diagnosis and treatment of CD in girls with ADHD. While the short-term response to stimulants is the same in these two groups, children with ADHD and conduct disorder have higher rates of antisocial personality as adults. To address this latter issue, additional professional intervention may be necessary.

EARLY SEXUAL ACTIVITY

We have known for some time that teenage girls with ADHD may be at greater risk for pregnancy than are other teenage girls.[27] This unfortunate situation may be true for a number of reasons. Teenage girls, who struggle with low self-esteem, as do many girls with ADHD, may seek affirmation through the sexual attentions of boys in an effort to compensate for feelings of inadequacy in other areas of their life. Furthermore, due to difficulties with impulse control, poor planning ability, and inconsistency, many of these girls are prone to have unprotected sex, use birth control inconsistently, and/or have multiple partners. As a result, these girls may be among the most at-risk for contracting a sexually transmitted disease or having an unwanted pregnancy during adolescence and young adulthood. In one follow-up study, young adults with ADHD were more likely than non-ADHD peers to become parents and to have been treated for sexually transmitted disease.[28]

Although risky sexual behavior and unplanned pregnancy are not typically examined as outcomes when ADHD is assessed using rating scales, they are risks associated with impulsivity. In a survey among teachers (grades eight and above), more reported to have observed promiscuous behavior in girls with ADHD than boys with the disorder.[29] In addition, a decreased likelihood of a partner's condom use was reported in a sample of female college undergraduates with ADHD, when compared to females without ADHD and males with ADHD.[30] However, this study did not report any differences in unplanned pregnancy rates between girls with and without ADHD, so additional data are needed to more clearly define the relationship between ADHD and the risk of unintended pregnancy in girls and women with ADHD. In contrast, another study found that higher ADHD symptom scores in young women were associated with an increased likelihood of several high-risk sexual behaviors, except inconsistent condom use, and the acquisition of sexually transmitted diseases.[31] A Finnish study found that girls with externalizing type of problems in childhood (e.g., conduct problems and hyperactivity) at age eight, have a significantly increased risk of becoming mothers before age 20.[32]

WHAT CAN PARENTS AND PROFESSIONALS DO TO HELP REDUCE THIS RISK?

- Support groups for girls with ADHD can help them feel more accepted and less alone, reducing their need to seek male sexual attention.

- Helping them become involved in structured, constructive activities will give them other outlets to develop self-esteem. Recent studies confirm what common sense tells us: adolescents who are kept busy in extracurricular activities, sports, church groups, and so on, are less likely to get in trouble during high school.

- An open, supportive relationship with their parents gives them somewhere to turn for advice if they do become sexually active — either to help them make a wise choice of birth control or to help make the best decision if they do become pregnant.

- Helping them find and develop islands of competence is highly beneficial. The girl who has many sources of support and self-esteem will be much less needy, and therefore, less vulnerable to sexual attention.

POOR DRIVING HABITS

Studies of teens with ADHD have shown that, in general, they have a greater likelihood of being involved in traffic accidents. One study reported that teens with ADHD had significantly more accidents. The researchers attributed this higher accident rate to problems with attention and cognitive control.[11] Most studies have only examined the driving behavior of boys with

ADHD, but one study in New Zealand [12] studied both boys and girls and found that girls with attention difficulties were at high risk for both traffic crashes and driving offenses.

The important message for parents is that their daughters with ADHD may need more practice in driving, so that driving skills become more automatic and require less concentrated effort and attention. Secondly, since attention problems seem to be strongly implicated in traffic accidents, girls (and boys) with ADHD should take care to drive in less distracting situations during their first years as a driver. They should avoid heavy traffic, social distractions, such as excited, talkative peers, and, it goes without saying, should never drink and drive. Teens with ADHD must maintain a more conscious awareness of their need to keep their eyes on the road.

In order to avoid accidents even in adulthood, individuals with ADHD may find themselves distracted by conversation while driving. For less experienced drivers, such a distraction could be all it takes to trigger a chain reaction leading to an accident. Thirdly, situations that may lead to impulsive reactions should be discussed in advance and avoided, if possible. Such situations might include driving with peers who are impulsive risk-takers, or who have been drinking and who may encourage a teenage girl with ADHD to take a risk for fun.

EMOTIONAL PROBLEMS AND MOOD DISORDERS

> *"I spent a lot of lonely times in my room. I look back on it now and believe that I suffered through depression during those years. I kept it so well-hidden, that my mom and dad never knew."* —Chris D.

Girls with ADHD have been found to have a 2.5 times higher risk for mood disorders (MD) as adolescents compared with girls without the disorder.[35] Mood disorder in these girls was associated with an earlier age at onset, a longer duration of symptoms (more than twice), more severe depression-associated impairment, a higher rate of suicidality, and a greater likelihood of requiring psychiatric hospitalization than mood disorders in girls without ADHD. Parental history of mood disorders and symptoms of mania were significant predictors of mood disorders among females with ADHD, independently of other predictors.

Parents and professionals need to be watchful during the teenage years to assess whether the normal emotional roller coaster for girls with ADHD has careened over the edge into a level of anxiety or depression that requires treatment in tandem with her treatment for ADHD. Emotions can tip quickly when environmental stresses suddenly overwhelm the teenage girl's already distressed system. An accidental pregnancy, the breakup of a relationship, a failed exam, a rejection letter from a college—any of these might be enough to push her into levels of anxiety or depression that may require both medication and psychotherapy or a psychiatric hospitalization.[35]

SUICIDE AND SELF-INJURY

Suicide attempts among girls with ADHD is a significant concern, but we are still attempting to understand exactly what factors may be related to suicide attempts. One study by Russell Barkley and his colleagues[36] showed that hyperactivity during childhood as well as the number of symptoms of conduct disorder were mild predictors of later suicide attempts in those with

ADHD. Another study included children with ADHD, mostly males, and none with the inattentive subtype, and found that these children were at greater risk for later suicide attempts compared to a comparison group.[37] Importantly, the girls included in this study were at greater risk of later depression or suicide attempts than were boys. Another study[38] found that poor emotional regulation was a strong predictor of self-injurious behavior. Considering the findings of these studies together, it appears that girls with ADHD and poor emotional regulation skills are those at higher risk for suicide attempts, and that hyperactivity and conduct disorder seem to somewhat increase that risk.

In the landmark studies of girls with and without ADHD, conducted by Hinshaw, girls with a childhood diagnosis of ADHD were followed into adolescence and young adulthood and found to have rates of psychiatric symptoms and functional impairments than the comparison group. When girls who were diagnosed with ADHD between seven and 12 years of age were followed up 10 years later, several negative patterns emerged. These patterns included the high occurrence of suicide attempts and self-injury in those with a diagnosis of combined type ADHD during their elementary school years.[39] ADHD in adolescent girls and young women carries a high risk of internalizing and externalizing disorders as well as impulsivity, so it is not unexpected that we find this increase in suicide attempts, and other self-injury behaviors. For girls with ADHD, consultation with a mental health professional for therapy and perhaps medication is clearly warranted.

Hinshaw then went on to examine which subgroups and which particularly features should serve as warning signs of suicidality for parents and professionals. In a follow-up study,[40] Hinshaw examined the possible pathways to self-harming behavior and suicide attempts among girls with ADHD. Findings revealed that women diagnosed in childhood with ADHD-C engaged in the most severe forms of non-suicide self-injury and experimented with the widest variety of methods relative to girls diagnosed with Inattentive ADHD and girls without ADHD. Although both ADHD subtypes engaged in more frequent self-injury than girls without ADHD, they did not significantly differ from each other.

Girls whose ADHD persisted were also found to have significantly higher reports of suicide attempts (22%) relative to girls without ADHD (4%). Externalizing behaviors (poor inhibition control and impulsiveness) at follow-up emerged as significant partial mediators of the ADHD-non-suicide self-injury severity link; internalizing symptoms during adolescence emerged as a significant partial mediator of the ADHD-suicide attempt.

As stated by the authors of this study, the above findings only underscore the importance of thorough and frequent monitoring of self-harmful behaviors among girls and young women with Combined type ADHD, particularly those with externalizing behaviors and persistent diagnostic profiles. Treatment to reduce impulsivity and internalizing behaviors may also help to reduce risk.

> *"I'm just not good at anything," Lisa, a ninth grade girl with ADHD, expressed despairingly. With regret and envy she described girls in her class who had made the cheerleading squad, earned top grades, or had already completed years of music or dance lessons, developing high levels of skill and self-confidence in the process. Lisa had taken up and dropped many interests—a pattern typical for girls with ADHD. At age 14, she no longer had*

faith in herself or in her capacity to stick with any endeavor. Easily discouraged, and with a low-frustration tolerance, she pursued each succeeding interest with less and less faith that she would discover a talent or develop a skill. Lisa became more withdrawn and agitated and was noted to begin to pluck at her eyelashes and eyebrows. Over a few months this escalated into pulling out the hairs on her thighs instead. Lisa's mother became concerned and brought her to a therapist when Lisa started saying that she wished she were dead and didn't know why she had ever been born.

WHAT CAN PARENTS DO TO CHANGE THIS NEGATIVE PROFILE

Parents can help their daughter with ADHD by encouraging her to discover and embrace her strengths rather than dwell on her weaknesses and failures. Girls who have developed ability or talent in some area seem to be much better inoculated against Lisa's cloud of self-defeating gloom. Teachers and parents may shrug off a girl's declaration that she has "no idea what she wants to do," reassuring her that most people don't figure that out until later. However, what they may not recognize is the particular vulnerability of girls with ADHD, who may have very little sense of accomplishment or ability. Rather than simply not having pinpointed a career path, these girls often suffer from a belief that they possess no valuable talent or ability.

One of the most constructive approaches in helping a girl with ADHD through her high school years is to actively help her develop and recognize areas of competence and talent. This is a first step toward helping her learn about herself and what types of post-high school training and employment would work well for her. It is important to consider not just her ADHD, but her abilities, interests, and personality as well. These girls often have a well-developed sense of what they're not good at, but very little awareness of their strengths. Awareness of strengths and abilities has a far greater value than its utilitarian value in career counseling. When girls with ADHD are in touch with their areas of competence, the less vulnerable they will be to the criticisms and frustrations that so often accompany ADHD.

The most therapeutic process for girls with ADHD is to begin to develop a sense of competence and ability through discovering islands of competence amidst the sea of challenges she faces during high school years. There are many arenas in which to do this, and exploration shouldn't be limited to career possibilities. Part-time work after school, even though it competes with study time, may give her a chance to feel capable, and to receive evidence of this in the form of a paycheck. Volunteering at a local hospital or nursing home, helping to build props for the school play, participating in a community beautification project, learning to ride horseback—these activities may not directly evolve into a career path, but can be enormously beneficial in helping her to build a sense of self-confidence.

EATING DISORDERS

Girls with ADHD can sometimes develop serious eating problems. Two follow-up studies of adolescent girls previously diagnosed with ADHD have found a significant incidence of eating disorders in this group.[41, 42] In the first study, girls with ADHD were found to be 3.6 times more likely to develop an eating disorder as girls without ADHD. Compared to girls without

ADHD, they were 5.6 times more likely to develop bulimia and 2.7 times more likely to develop anorexia nervosa. In the second study, it was found that the presence of impulsivity and the diagnosis of combined type ADHD best predicted adolescent eating abnormalities. In addition, peer rejection and parent-child relationship patterns were seen as predictive of eating disorders in girls with ADHD.

Addressing these serious eating problems while treating the accompanying ADHD with stimulants to decrease impulsivity may decrease the urge to binge quite effectively.[43] These girls tend to binge, and once they begin eating they have difficulty stopping, impulsively eating everything in sight, even when they are not hungry. Stimulant medication helps these girls stop and think before eating, and decreases their appetites if they tend to overeat.

For girls with ADHD who are also picky eaters and have difficulty with food textures, stimulant medication may complicate the picture by decreasing their appetite. Serving preferred foods and increasing or supplementing caloric intake may be necessary as part of the treatment for this group. For girls who are overweight because of eating too much or not knowing when to stop, the side effect of decreased appetite in addition to improved attention and decreased impulsivity can be used to their advantage. Under supervision, with a structured plan, appropriate weight loss may be achieved. A related concern, however, is the girl who abuses medication and its side effects to lose weight. All individuals, male or female, should have regular follow-ups with the prescribing physician, including height and weight checks. Possible side effects should always be discussed, and weight loss issues may need to be addressed, if this seems to be a problem. Additional counseling or referrals to a nutritionist and mental health professional may be necessary in such cases.

SUBSTANCE ABUSE AND OTHER ADDICTIVE BEHAVIORS

In general, adolescents with ADHD are at an increased risk for substance use, but the pathways through which this risk emerges are not sufficiently understood. In one recent study,[44] tobacco, alcohol, and marijuana use outcomes were compared between adolescents diagnosed with ADHD in early childhood and demographically similar controls. Participants were assessed from age five until age 18. A comprehensive history of adolescent substance use was compiled for each participant. Results indicated that when compared with controls, adolescents with ADHD were more likely to try cigarettes, initiate alcohol use at early ages, and smoke marijuana more frequently. Furthermore, adolescents with ADHD were four to five times more likely than controls to escalate to heavy cigarette and marijuana use after trying these substances once. Adolescents with ADHD who escalated to heavy use patterns were more likely to display early cigarette use and marked problems with family members, but displayed fewer peer problems. Furthermore, severe ADHD symptoms accounted for an increase in Conduct Disorder (CD), and subsequently, escalating CD symptoms in childhood were viewed as a mediator of the relationship between ADHD and cigarette and marijuana use. Maternal drinking during their childhood was seen as the strongest predictor of later adolescent alcohol use.

Risks, of course, continue and intensify as an increasing number of peers are involved in smoking cigarettes, drinking alcohol, smoking marijuana, and experimenting with a range of other drugs. Adolescent girls with ADHD diagnosed before the age of 12 years seem to be at great risk,[45] with another study reporting that 14% of girls with ADHD have a substance use disorder, and one in five smoke cigarettes.[46] As teens with ADHD reach age 16 or 17 and obtain their driver's licenses, the dangers associated with drinking and drugs increase greatly. Parents who are concerned about the possibility of impulsive drinking and driving should very carefully consider whether the convenience of having a teen that can transport herself is worth the potentially lethal results of combining drugs or alcohol and driving.

DEVELOPING LIFE MANAGEMENT SKILLS

High school is a time to gradually separate from the dominance and control of parents. But this transition is often intensified and prolonged when ADHD is in the picture. Along with the normal impulses toward independence, comes a gnawing, rarely expressed fear that she can't really handle the responsibility and expectations of self-reliance that accompany her growing freedom. This combination can make the high school years an exceptionally bumpy ride, as teenage girls with ADHD demand more independence only to feel over-whelmed, even frightened, by the dilemmas created as a result of their impulsivity, disorganization, and poor planning.

If your daughter is the quiet, daydreamy type, she may engage in less of the behavior that can be so frightening for parents — defying parental rules, drinking, experimenting with drugs, or early sexual behavior, but these years are still likely to be fraught with pain for her. Many quiet, shy young women with ADHD report having felt too intimidated to practice the skills needed to be self-sufficient when they leave home.

Parents can help their daughters gain skills for autonomy and independence by remaining patient, and by recognizing that the process may take their daughter with ADHD longer than the average adolescent. Advance practice can be helpful. Here are some suggestions.

- If she hopes to go away from home to college, she may benefit greatly by attending a school that offers an extended orientation period in the summer before freshman year for students who have special needs.

- It may be very helpful to open a checking account during high school, where she can deposit any cash gifts or money earned from summer jobs. In this fashion, she has a longer period of time to learn the habit of recording checks and keeping an accurate account balance.

- Learning to handle charge cards responsibly is crucial to adult life, but can be very difficult for any teen. Obtaining a card with a very low limit — $200-$300 — can provide experience without opening the door to disaster.

- Providing her with a clothing allowance during high school also can give her experience in managing money, setting priorities, and making decisions within defined limits.

- Learning to use a day planner is one of the most critical skills your daughter needs to master as she leaves home for college or the working world. A day planner is not only for recording appointments, but for recording all crucial information — phone numbers, addresses, shopping lists, directions, and so on.

- By developing the habit of writing all-important information in one place, she will have a skill that is invaluable for managing ADHD tendencies toward forgetfulness and disorganization.

- The simple act of setting an alarm clock and depending upon oneself to get up on time in the morning is often very challenging for girls with ADHD. This is a skill best practiced at home, where parents can remain a back-up system, rather than waiting until she is away at college or in her first apartment.

- Working with a coach who specializes in ADHD can often be helpful for girls as they learn to organize and prioritize. All students face increasing, multiple demands as they enter their high school years—multiple teachers and assignments, extracurricular activities, part-time jobs, increased responsibilities to help at home, learning to drive, beginning to date—the list is long and daunting. Girls with ADHD will need help in organizing and managing these multiple demands, and in making ADHD-friendly choices so that they are not juggling more than they can manage.

Reinforcing assertiveness and self-advocacy skills

Saying "No" is not typically included in the set of tools we equip our girls with. Rather, they are taught to be cooperative, compliant, and helpful. Many girls with ADHD try to fade into the woodwork, fearing any interaction that may call upon them to be assertive. Sari Solden writes extensively in her book, *Women with Attention Deficit Disorder*, about the difficulty that most women with ADHD have in being appropriately assertive in expressing their needs for assistance or accommodation.[47] Those girls whose ADHD is more external, like many boys with ADHD, may say "no" frequently, but may not do so with diplomacy and grace, resulting in their being labeled as having an attitude or worse.

The difficulty of learning to advocate for needs related to ADHD compounds the assertiveness challenge for a girl. Added to the self-consciousness and self-doubts that any teen with ADHD might experience when they first attempt to express their needs, girls have the extra burden of having been trained since their earliest years to compromise, comply, and not be bossy or demanding.

> *"I remember my mother always saying to me in elementary school and high school that I shouldn't be so difficult, so bossy. She'd tell me that I wouldn't have any friends and the teachers wouldn't like me if I didn't try harder to be 'nice'."* — Cara

During her high school years a girl needs to develop the self-advocacy skills required for more independent life beyond high school — whether in an educational setting or in the workforce. She will have to express herself confidently and convincingly to professors or employers who are ill-informed about ADHD. Parental validation of her right to express her opinion, and help in learning to express it in a constructive, effective manner are critical for success in development of these skills.

High schools often stress the need for students with ADHD to become their own self-advocates rather than continue to rely on parents. However, few high schools provide help in learning these crucial skills. This is another area where a girls' ADHD support group can provide enormous benefit. In this setting, girls can practice these skills using role-play, receive support when they feel intimidated or embarrassed in their efforts, and strategize the best ways to explain and assert their needs.

Coaching and the benefits of structure

As with girls of all ages with ADHD, teenage girls need support, encouragement, and structure. Because teenage girls are trying to develop skills necessary for independence, sometimes it is more helpful when someone other than their parents provides structure and fosters accountability. This could be a therapist, coach, or school guidance counselor.

Coaching can be helpful at younger ages, but as the girls with ADHD enter high school, coaching may be a key element in their efforts to learn to meet the greatly increased demands for organization and planning. It is critical for a teenage girl to collaborate with her coach rather than feeling that the coach is just one more adult in her life who instructs and restricts her. Good rapport between the coach and teen is essential. Parents need to take a more backseat role, allowing their teenage daughter, together with the coach, to set the agenda. Working with a coach throughout high school can help a teenage girl with ADHD construct a critical bridge between childhood dependence and the need for increasing independence as she leaves home for college or the work world in a few short years. These are the years when the teenage girl needs to learn the importance of being on time, staying organized, and setting priorities rather than staying in a reactive mode. Working with a coach will allow her to see that these skills are all goals she can set for herself as opposed to ones set by her parents.

College placement counseling

As the teenage girl with ADHD approaches her junior year of high school, she and her family should be working together very actively to make good decisions regarding what she will do after high school. The assistance of a specialized college placement counselor can be especially useful to help her and her parents sort through the maze of possibilities: community college, vocational training, attending a four-year college while remaining at home, going away to a small college, or applying to a large university. Not only is there a wide variety of educational settings to choose from, but there is also a wide range in the degree of support available for students with ADHD at various educational institutions.

The most critical element in the decision-making process is to accurately assess her level of maturity, her readiness to leave the structure and security of home, her need for academic support, and her preferences regarding the atmosphere, geographic location, and courses of study offered by various schools. This daunting process should not be left for the teenage girl with ADHD to address alone. However, she should be an active participant, expressing her preferences and desires, and taking part in visiting, interviewing, and considering her options.

Most teens with ADHD need considerable support when faced with the formidable task of writing college essays, asking for letters of recommendation, and completing application forms.

Because tension often runs high between parents and teens around this process, primary support is sometimes best provided by a coach or tutor. The fact that a girl procrastinates and postpones the daunting process of choosing and applying to colleges should not be interpreted by parents as a sign that she is not ready for college. It is exactly these types of detailed administrative tasks that are difficult for her, and may never be an area of strength. Many girls with ADHD benefit greatly from working with a coach or tutor that can shepherd them through the process of writing college essays, completing applications, and requesting letters of recommendation.

Career counseling/ability testing

The latest statistics still show that women, at all educational levels, earn less than men with the same level of training. Social stereotypes continue to strongly influence not only the hiring practices of employers, but also the career choices that young women pursue. Typically, many of the jobs performed by women involve caring for, supporting, or administratively assisting others. Often, it is just these sorts of jobs that are particularly unsuitable for women with ADHD because they involve being the support system for others, rather than allowing them to build a support system around themselves. The very tasks of reminding, attending to details, organizing, and assisting with paperwork are the tasks that are typically the least-suited to the ADHD brain.

> *"When I graduated from high school, I didn't have a clue as to what my interests or strong points were. I did end up going to a community college, taking secretarial classes. But after going there for two years, I decided that it was too boring. I was the only one in the family who*

didn't know what they wanted to do. I just didn't seem to have any ambition. After college, I got the idea that I wanted to be a hairdresser, so I went to a beauty school. I remember my dad saying, 'I'll pay for it as long as you get a job out of it.' I said I would. I got a job, but I hated it. I was so bad at it I quit. I couldn't keep up with the pace and I just lost interest. I really felt like a failure. To this day I don't know what kind of job would be good for me."
— A 29-year-old with ADHD, who is now seeking career guidance.

During high school, girls with ADHD need to be educated about ADHD-friendly jobs and work environments so that their career selections and job paths are not ill-chosen. Assessment of high school girls with ADHD should include career interest and ability testing, as well as the Myers-Briggs Type Inventory to help them understand core personality traits and values that are so important to match with their chosen career path. Such tests can become the basis of helping them identify strengths and talents, and can be of enormous value in helping them make good choices of jobs or of courses of study in college. Without this kind of assistance and guidance, many young women with ADHD will experience repeated failure and frustration as they move from one inappropriate career path to the next.

Although recent research confirms the chronic nature of the symptoms and impairments associated with ADHD for girls, a sizable minority were found to be doing well in adulthood despite their childhood ADHD. It is thus important to remember that although a childhood diagnosis of ADHD portends continuing difficulty, such outcomes are by no means inevitable and there is much we can do to help these girls develop into strong, independent, young women despite their ADHD.

CONCLUSION

The high school years are among the most challenging for any teen, but can be especially difficult for girls with ADHD. To bridge the challenges of high school, they need support from peers, parents, and schools, combined with appropriate treatment programs that meet their particular needs and issues. With these supports and interventions, girls with ADHD will be able to make the crucial transition from the chaos and self-doubt of adolescence to a sense of growing strength, efficacy, and competence as they enter their young adult years.

QUESTIONS TO ASK YOURSELF ABOUT YOUR HIGH SCHOOL DAUGHTER

This list is designed to aid parents who may have questions about the possibility of ADHD in their teenage daughter. We ask you to think about your daughter as you answer the following questions. Some signs of ADHD in teens can be confusing because they may be behaviors typical of all teens, but are perhaps more marked in teens with ADHD. It may be helpful to look at the questions for parents of middle school, elementary school, and preschool daughters and answer them retrospectively, looking back at your daughter's behavior at younger ages. Keep in mind, however, that many girls do not exhibit obvious signs of ADHD in their younger years. You should not rule out the possibility of ADHD if your daughter seems to exhibit signs now, but did not exhibit them earlier. Even though you may answer "Yes" to many of the following questions, this does not necessarily indicate that your daughter has ADHD, but if your concerns are aroused, it may be advisable to seek a professional evaluation.

- Does she have great difficulty in planning and organizing long-term assignments?
- Does she have a strong tendency to procrastinate?
- Does she tend to study and/or write papers at the last minute, possibly staying up all night?
- Does she seem flighty or scattered?
- Does she have trouble getting to sleep at night and waking in the morning?
- Does she leave a trail of belongings in every room she passes through?
- Does she frequently misplace keys, umbrellas, cell phones and other personal belongings?

- Does she seem overwhelmed by school?
- Is she hypertalkative?
- Does she frequently interrupt in conversation?
- Do her emotional reactions, both positive and negative, seem out of proportion to the event?
- Does she appear to have difficulty with anxiety or depression?
- Do you feel that her academic achievement is significantly below her intellectual potential?
- Does she need to work in a rigid, almost compulsive fashion for long hours to complete her work?
- Does she work hard for teachers she likes, but very little for teachers she dislikes?
- Does she have a pattern of starting out well, but of losing steam as the school year progresses?
- Is she often late?
- Is she forgetful and/or absentminded?
- Are you concerned about her judgment regarding drinking, driving, and sexual activity?
- Are you concerned about drug experimentation or abuse?
- Does she have low frustration tolerance?
- Does she frequently forget important items at home or at school?
- Does she seem to have an exceptionally difficult time in the week(s) prior to her period?
- Does she smoke cigarettes?
- Does she drink large quantities of caffeinated drinks?
- Does she engage in binge eating or have difficulty with her weight or body image?
- Does she tend to quickly lose interest and drop hobbies, interests, and other activities?

- Does she have difficulty developing and sticking to routines?
- Do some of her behaviors seem overly rigid or compulsive?
- Does she seem stressed much of the time?

CHAPTER SEVEN

Common Developmental Issues

ADHD IS A DEVELOPMENTAL DISORDER that commonly co-occurs with other developmental disorders. Suspicion of a developmental disorder may require a consultation or assessment by a specialist in these areas, since misdiagnosis does occur. Sometimes the underachievement of a girl with ADHD is complicated by a developmental disorder in one or more of the following areas: auditory processing, visual processing, sensory integration, memory, motor coordination, or visual-motor integration, autism and Tourette syndrome. In addition, learning disorders in the areas of reading, writing, or math are also commonly associated with ADHD.

In this chapter, we will briefly describe associated developmental/learning disorders. Some of these disorders have many symptoms that overlap with those of ADHD. Very careful assessment by specialists including speech/language specialists, occupational therapists, and neuropsychologists may be in order to sort out exactly what is going on with an individual girl, so that appropriate treatment and/or academic accommodations and supports can be put in place.

DEVELOPMENTAL COORDINATION DISORDER (DCD)

DCD is a clinical term used to refer to what the general public might call physical awkwardness or clumsiness. Approximately 1/3 of children with ADHD have developmental coordination disorder (DCD).[1] Girls with DCD have difficulty with motor planning, with balance, and with monitoring their movement through space. DCD problems become more challenging as motor skills increase in importance in elementary school, however, they can also create challenges in preschool, making girls with DCD less able to engage in play with their peers and more hesitant to try new skills that involve a motor component. In this way DCD can contribute to hesitance and low self-esteem.

Both fine and gross motor difficulties may become more problematic for a girl when her peers have more advanced motor development. Girls with gross motor problems may avoid bike riding or roller-skating with friends. Children with predominantly inattentive presentation ADHD tend to be more affected than those at the hyperactive/impulsive end of the ADHD continuum. Girls and boys are equally affected by motor problems.[2]

Girls with fine motor coordination problems may have difficulty buttoning and zipping clothing; may have difficulty learning to tie shoelaces, typically have difficulty with handwriting as they enter school, and are much less adept than age mates at drawing and coloring. Some parents and teachers mistake fine motor problems for "not trying," adding insult to injury for a child that is unable to perform these tasks.

As girls with motor problems enter elementary school years, they may experience embarrassment in physical education classes as they are not able to perform at the same level as peers. They may have difficulty with the fine motor skills required by popular girls' activities such as stringing tiny beads on wires to make costume jewelry or braiding strands of cord to make bracelets.

It is important for parents of girls with ADHD to be sensitive to both fine and gross motor coordination problems because these issues affect many aspects of daily life and can lead to frustration, embarrassment, and lowered self-esteem when a girl is unable to perform the tasks that age mates are routinely performing.

CENTRAL AUDITORY PROCESSING DISORDER (CAPD)

It has long been known that up to 50% of children with central auditory processing disorder (CAPD) also have ADHD.[3] Processing verbal information requires a complex set of skills including auditory acuity, sound discrimination, auditory memory, and synthesis of the meaning of the words expressed. A parent might begin to suspect auditory processing problems if a daughter has difficulty understanding what is said to her, if she responds inappropriately to what was said, or if she responds very slowly when spoken to. Before exploring an auditory processing problem, a complete hearing test is indicated to rule out any contributing physiological factors. It is important to remember that slow auditory-processing can reflect the distraction of ADHD as much as it can a true auditory processing disorder. There is tremendous overlap in the symptoms of CAPD and ADHD and careful differential diagnosis must be made by a speech pathologist if CAPD is suspected.[4]

SPEECH AND LANGUAGE PROBLEMS

ADHD girls are more likely to manifest speech and language problems than are their peers without ADHD.[5] Often, the developmental history taken from the parents reveals that the onset of speech was significantly delayed. More than half of language-based disorders originate from poor attentional control during early development, as well as from a decreased ability to lock language into long-term memory. Since expressive language problems are far more likely than receptive language problems, it is not surprising that the capacity of a girl with ADHD to use language as a way of guiding her behavior and controlling her impulses is limited. While language-based difficulties do respond to remediation, determining if there is a true impairment of skills in addition to the obstacles posed by ADHD is the first step.

TIC DISORDERS

About 50-60 % of children with Tourette syndrome also have ADHD, while a minority of ADHD children also have a motor or vocal tic. Only about one in five children with Tourette syndrome are female.[6,7] A child with ADHD and Tourette syndrome has a greater likelihood of developing other conditions, including anxiety, intermittent explosive disorder, and other emotional regulation problems.[8]

AUTISM SPECTRUM DISORDER/ASPERGER'S SYNDROME

Until the publication of the DSM-5 in 2013,[9] a distinction was made between Asperger's syndrome and autism. Now, we refer to the autism spectrum disorder (ASD). Children that would formerly be labeled with Asperger's are now referred to as having high-functioning autism. Although Asperger's is no longer an official diagnosis, we mention it here because many parents of girls have come to understand and describe their daughters using this label. A sudden change to the term autism, which heretofore referred to individuals with more severe intellectual and social impairments, may feel jarring to some parents.

Similar to the history of ADHD, whose symptoms were developed through the observation of boys, autism spectrum disorder (ASD) symptoms have also been derived through observation of an almost entirely male population, which can result in a self-reinforcing finding that more boys than girls have ASD (or ADHD).[10] Recently, the Autism Spectrum Symptom Questionnaire was revised and extended to include items that were better at capturing the female ASD phenotype.[11] This is a new and growing area of research interest. At this point, several authors suggest that because females with ASD have a stronger social drive, their symptoms may be more subtle than those of boys. On the revised questionnaires, several items emerged that appear to be more typical of girls with ADHD, including:

1. Avoids demands
2. Very determined
3. Careless with physical appearance and dress
4. Interacts mostly with younger children

It has been speculated that girls with ASD tend to avoid direct demands from others because the demands engender anxiety, whereas behaving according to internal decisions allows them to feel more control over their environment. These girls were more likely to simply ignore demands rather than to actively resist them. They had a much stronger pattern of preferring to interact with younger children than did boys. Again, researchers speculate that with younger children these girls can satisfy their needs for social interaction while maintaining control of decisions during play. Girls were not as likely as boys to engage in the classic pattern of repetitive behaviors. A study of girls and boys with ASD, who were not intellectually impaired and with no clear comorbid disorder, showed subclinical patterns of depressive disorder, anxiety separation disorder, agoraphobia and specific phobias, obsessive compulsive disorder (OCD), and attention deficit hyperactivity disorder (ADHD).[12] Due to these numerous subclinical disorders found in children with autism, it is likely that one or more of these will rise to the level of a true disorder as these children age.

There is evidence that girls exhibiting signs of autism and ADHD tend to be overlooked or misidentified.[13] Girls with autism frequently had ADHD as well as other disorders including anxiety, depression, learning problems and social behavioral problems. These girls reported being bullied and trying to avoid participation in athletic activities where such bullying often took place. Peers viewed these girls as different, awkward, and vulnerable. When a girl's social problems go beyond shyness or a lack of awareness of her impact on others (traits common among girls with ADHD), it may be advisable to have her carefully assessed by a professional who is expert in both ADHD and autism spectrum disorder.

LEARNING DISORDERS

A significant number of girls with ADHD have some type of learning disorder. Studies have shown that about 70% of children with ADHD also have a learning disorder, with a learning disorder in written expression two times more common (65%) than a learning disorder in reading, math, or spelling.[14] Even for the brightest girls with ADHD, school can be a painful journey of underachievement. Much of their psychic energy is directed toward hiding their differences, leaving less energy to devote to required and leisure-time activities. They live with a pervasive sense of confusion and embarrassment. They know they are smart enough to be on top of things yet they mysteriously underachieve, even when they are trying their hardest. This undermining pattern could make even the most confident student doubt herself.

Learning disorders may appear to emerge during these middle school years among bright/gifted girls with ADHD because their native intelligence allowed them to compensate. As the demands for reading, writing, productivity, and memory grow, bright middle school and high school girls with ADHD may be diagnosed with one or more learning disorders for the first time.

Reading

According to one recent review, reading disorder (RD), also referred to as dyslexia, coexists with ADHD in 33% to 45% of cases.[15] Reading comprehension is a different skill than simple word decoding. A student may have excellent word-attack skills and word recognition skills, but still struggle with reading comprehension. It is also true that some bright students with poorly developed decoding skills can develop rather strong reading comprehension skills through using contextual clues to comprehend meaning. It is generally agreed that reading comprehension involves a complex interaction of variables including the reader herself, the reader's interest in the topic, the knowledge the reader has of the topic, the reading strategies the reader employs, the complexity of the text material, and the concentration level of the reader. Girls with predominantly inattentive ADHD are more likely to have a reading disorder than girls with combined or hyperactive/impulsive presentation ADHD.[16] When parents suspect a reading problem, they should schedule a complete visual exam for their daughter to rule out vision problems.

Even without a reading disorder, reading can be incredibly difficult for many children with ADHD, especially if the content is not inherently interesting. If a girl with ADHD resists reading, reads slowly, and rarely reads for pleasure, a psychoeducational assessment can help determine whether she has a true reading disorder, or whether her struggles are related to inattention and distractibility.

Reading difficulties are not alike for all girls with ADHD. Some reread the same passage repeatedly, struggling to stay focused. Some girls can hyperfocus for a couple of pages before they begin to skim, and then fall asleep from the effort. Others may read quickly and superficially so that they have little comprehension, but can say they are done. Some can only read in brief spurts, prefering the *Newsweek* approach to current events — photos with catchy captions and a paragraph summarizing the issue. The only thing overtly noticeable to a teacher or parent is that these girls appear to read extremely slowly. The adults are then left to their own devices to interpret what they see.

Writing

A child is considered to have a written language disorder (also called a Disorder of Written Expression) if her writing skills fall significantly below what would be expected, given her age, IQ, and appropriate instruction in spelling and writing. The likelihood that a child with ADHD has a written language disorder is greater than 65%, and when reading disorder is also present, the likelihood rises to 95%.[17] Parents and teachers need to be aware of this very high risk and should automatically consider the presence of a writing disorder when a girl with ADHD demonstrates reading difficulties.

The term dysgraphia has been used in the past to refer to writing difficulties. This term can be confusing because it refers to all aspects of writing from the physical mechanics of handwriting, being able to form legible letters, to the spacing between words and between lines of words, to spelling, as well as to the more complex task of the organization and coherent expression of thoughts. Word retrieval, often a difficulty for girls with ADHD, also plays a frustrating role when they are attempting to write.

The act of writing is a veritable minefield for many girls with ADHD — poor fine motor skills and difficulty persisting in motor activities make the physical act of writing uncomfortable. She may use too much pencil pressure, making her fingers ache with cramps and fatigue. The great discrepancy between the speed of her thoughts and the speed at which she can write makes her either leave out words or sentences, or forget some of her ideas while she struggles to print. Difficulty organizing her thoughts and problems with word retrieval make initiation of the writing assignment torturous. Finally, proofreading is too tedious for most girls with ADHD; they can hyperfocus for a little while, but then they'll lose motivation to finish.

The demand for writing continually ramps up from grade school through high school. Written expression problems may be more common among students with ADHD because a great many executive functions are required to write a good paper. A research paper requires organization, long-term planning, prolonged motivation, and consistent self-monitoring in order to work within the paradigm of a research paper.

EXECUTIVE FUNCTIONING DISORDERS

Executive functioning (EF) skills are the higher order cognitive skills that allow us to succeed in planning and carrying out a task. EF functions include the ability to plan, organize, self-monitor, control impulses, moderate emotional responses, and to focus, shift and sustain our attention. Executive functioning skills are complex and so critical to overall functioning and success that we have developed a separate chapter to this topic — Chapter Eight.

Parents will be encouraged to learn that a recent study of females with ADHD from childhood through young adulthood show that EF skills significantly improve, accompanied by a decrease in ADHD symptoms.[18] It is believed that this improvement is due to the continued maturation of the prefrontal cortex of the brain, the area of the brain where these higher level cognitive functions take place, and the last area of the brain to fully mature. ADHD coaching primarily focuses on the development of executive functions such as time management, task management, planning, and prioritizing.

CONCLUSION

It's important that parents of girls with ADHD (as well as the girls themselves) do not overreact to the presence of multiple diagnoses. All of these different labels have more to do with the current state of our diagnostic system than a reflection of so many things being wrong in an individual girl. In fact, all of these developmental issues show a great deal of overlap. What's important is that parents and girls with ADHD develop a clear understanding of both strengths and weaknesses. From there, the task becomes to build a life that allows for a girl with ADHD to function primarily from her areas of strength, to work on improving areas of weakness, while receiving the supports she needs to succeed when she is required to function in areas of relative weakness.

CHAPTER EIGHT

Executive Functioning Skills
Keys to Success

WHAT ARE EXECUTIVE FUNCTIONING (EF) SKILLS?

Executive functioning (EF) skills can be thought of as the cognitive skills that are needed to accomplish goals. A recent study by Barkley,[1] analyzing responses to his Deficits in Executive Functioning Scale (DEFS), found that EF skills tend to group into five factors:

1. Time management
2. Organization and problem-solving
3. Self-discipline
4. Motivation
5. Emotional regulation

ADHD symptoms are generally consistent with difficulties in all of these EF skills. Many believe that good EF skills are even more critical than intelligence for success in adult life.[2] Before focusing specifically on how girls with ADHD are impacted by EF challenges, let's look at EF skills as they develop from childhood into adolescence and beyond.

EF SKILLS START TO APPEAR EARLY

Normal development of attention and self-control begins in earliest childhood. One attentional system is involved in orienting and exploring the immediate environment, driven by novelty. We are all familiar with the incessant energy and curiosity of infants and toddlers to explore their world. When only this attention system is online, a child is easy to distract from an undesirable activity by simply providing a novel, interesting stimulation. "Look at the birdie!"

By age three or four, a second attentional system comes online, which involves higher-level controls.[3] This is the beginning of the development of executive functions. Preschoolers start to develop self-control. This control is assisted by language acquisition that allows self-talk which the child can use to maintain motivation, persistence, following multistep directions, and motor responses. These skills are supported by the ongoing maturation of the prefrontal areas of the brain where executive functions are supported. The prefrontal area is one significant part of the brain that is impacted by ADHD. The good news is that the prefrontal area of the brain continues to develop until we are in our mid-to-late twenties. See Chapter Two for a more in-depth discussion of the prefrontal cortex (PFC).

DEVELOPMENT OF EF SKILLS OVER TIME

During childhood, parents and other adults tend to serve as external prefrontal lobes, providing constant support for their child's EF skills, not letting a child stay up too late, eat ice cream for breakfast, or forget to leave for school on time. However, some executive functions begin to emerge even in preschool years. Ideally, as a child matures there is an age-appropriate reduction of external support in step with a child's strengthening of EF abilities.

Preschool years

Throughout the day, at preschool and at home we teach preschoolers EF skills: "Take turns" (impulse control); "Use your words, not your hands!" (emotional regulation); "Use your inside voice." (self-monitoring); "Remember what we do to get ready for bed?" (planning skills).

In the famous marshmallow study by Walter Mischel and colleagues [4] at Stanford University, preschool children were placed in a room sitting in a chair with a marshmallow placed on the table in front of them. The room was deliberately unstimulating. The examiner told the child that the marshmallow was for them and that they could eat it at any time, but if they waited until after the examiner returned to the room they could have a second marshmallow. The examiner then left the room and observed the child's behavior. Some ate the marshmallow immediately, while others were able to wait the full 15-minute interval and earned a second marshmallow. When these preschool participants were followed up forty years later, there was a distinct advantage among the children who had been able to wait. Those with the self-control to delay gratification had higher educational levels and higher incomes than their more impulsive counterparts.

A great deal of attention has been paid recently, to the idea of teaching EF skills to preschoolers, with the idea that although some children may have an inherent advantage in EF skills (those that waited for the second marshmallow), that EF skills can be taught and strengthened. The Tools of the Mind programs,[5] based on Vigotsky's theory that children can learn EF skills through structured role-playing games,[6] have been instituted in a number of public and private preschools nationwide. EF skills are then integrated into the standard school curriculum with supports and scaffolding that are gradually removed as a child shows that she has internalized a particular skill. For example, a child with difficulty listening is given a large picture of an ear as an external reminder to listen; a girl who has difficulty sitting in her assigned place on the rug is given a specific *spot* on the rug with her name on it, and then holds hands with her classmates on either side. This scaffolding is removed when she is able to sit in her assigned place throughout the activity. Montessori schools, although they do not directly refer to executive functioning skills, engage each child in multiple activities that reinforce EF skills.[7]

Ability to delay gratification (waiting to get two marshmallows instead of settling for one) is a critical life skill. But to be able to delay gratification is related to other factors, such as the ability to remove oneself from temptations, to think long-term and measure immediate gain against long-term gain, as well as the confidence that one can succeed at a long-term effort. Parents begin to teach delay of gratification by requiring children to wait for dinner rather than snacking a half-hour before the meal. Waiting for one's turn in a game teaches a child the ability to delay gratification. And putting nickels or quarters in a piggy bank in order to save up for a coveted toy or game is a powerful lesson in delay of gratification that children can begin to learn at an early age.

Elementary school years

During elementary school there is a gradual shift both at home and at school to more self-initiated routines, including morning routines, homework routines, chore routines, and bedtime routines. Children can benefit greatly from external *scaffolding* (supports) as they develop these more demanding EF skills. For example, a child can follow a routine more easily when given a chart to reference and check off items as they are completed. Becoming more time aware is a very important EF skill. Parents can provide scaffolding for time awareness using a timer with an audible countdown.

Persistence is an important EF skill to work on during elementary school years. Often, the best scaffolding is simply the presence of a parent or other adult while a task that requires persistence is underway. Greater physical self-control develops during these early childhood years — staying seated during a meal, standing in line while waiting, and keeping hands to oneself. Planning skills begin to develop as a child joins in projects at school, at home, and during group social activities.

Girls with ADHD often begin to exhibit signs of anxiety as the demands for EF skills increase in elementary school. They fear being in trouble with the teacher if they forget to bring standard supplies to school, or forget to hand in a homework assignment. Parents may heighten a girl's anxiety by expressing frustration that their daughter left her jacket at school or forgot to bring home a book necessary for homework.

Learning from natural consequences is often ineffective for those girls with ADHD and poor executive functioning. Not being able to participate in physical education because a girl forgot her gym clothes will rarely result in remembering her gym clothes next time. It's not a lack of motivation, but rather a lack of adequate prospective memory (remembering to do something at some future point in time), a lack of organizational skills and poor planning skills.

Middle school years

During middle school years, demands for EF skills greatly increase while scaffolding at school decreases. Many children with ADHD who have coped reasonably well during elementary school begin to show strain and feelings of overwhelm during middle school. A middle school student has many teachers, a complicated schedule, and multiple homework assignments. She has more long-term assignments that require planning and persistence. A parent needs to be sensitive to the level of scaffolding needed by their particular child. Encouragement, support, and structure are important as she learns to operate more independently, to become more aware of the need to manage her time, and to plan and execute long-term projects.

High school years

In high school, the EF demands continue to escalate. Grades take on greater importance as they will be considered by colleges to which a student applies. Homework assignments increase in length and complexity, along with the planning and organizational demands that result from participation in other activities such as sports, clubs, and part-time jobs.

DO GIRLS WITH ADHD EXPERIENCE EF CHALLENGES DIFFERENTLY THAN BOYS?

All children with ADHD have EF challenges, but social expectations of EF skills for boys and girls are often quite different. Let's consider how our expectations for girls differ from expectations for boys and how EF challenges affect a girl's ability to live up to those expectations.

EF SKILLS AND GIRLS' SOCIAL INTERACTION PATTERNS

While boys are expected to be rough and tumble, competitive and risk-taking, girls are expected, from a very young age, to be more self-controlled and more tuned in to the needs and feelings of others. If we observe girls' interactions we will notice that they are generally more collaborative and communicative than boys. Among boys it is more typical to focus on a joint activity rather than on feelings and reactions and interactions. Competition is expected, and aggression, verbal or physical, is more tolerated among boys, if not encouraged.

The social interactions typical of girls depend upon an array of good EF skills. If we examine girls' social interactions, it becomes clear that the abilities to plan a response in the midst of a social interaction, to inhibit an undesirable response, to recall what was said in earlier conversations, to organize and initiate social interactions with others, and to inhibit interruptions during conversations while holding future comments in working memory are all critical to positive social interactions.

These EF skills are basic to a stable network of friendships, in which it is important to be aware of the perspective of others, to engage in behaviors that are prosocial in nature rather than simply serving one's own immediate needs, and will all lead to greater peer acceptance in adolescence and later. Self-control is required because social interactions among girls are typically collaborative rather than competitive. Collaboration requires give and take, attention to multiple social cues, verbal and non-verbal, and good emotional regulation. The EF skills expected in girls' social interactions prove very challenging for many girls with ADHD.

Dr. Stephen Hinshaw at UC Berkeley has spent many years studying the social skills of girls with ADHD and how these girls are perceived by girls without ADHD. While some girls with ADHD are very socially successful, Hinshaw has found that most girls with ADHD struggle to fit in. Some girls are seen as too loud or insistent, while girls that are shy and less verbal remain at the sidelines, ignored by more verbally skilled peers.[8, 9] Hyperactive/impulsive girls may be socially rejected while shy, inattentive girls are socially neglected.

SUGAR AND SPICE AND EVERYTHING NICE

Another significant gender difference has to do with personal grooming. Girls are praised for looking pretty while scraped knees and grass stains are standard issue for boys. Expectations regarding girls' grooming and clothing have certainly relaxed in recent years, but girls continue to spend extensive time styling their hair, applying make-up, and watching each other carefully to take note of the latest fashion trends.

As the author of *What I Wish my Mother had Known* (Chapter One) related, she, and many other girls with ADHD, have difficulty maintaining the careful grooming standards of their peers. Hair becomes tousled, nail polish chipped, shoes muddied or tights torn. Once again, to meet the standards expected of girls, careful attention and self-control are required, two traits often in short supply among girls with ADHD.

HOW CAN PARENTS HELP THEIR DAUGHTERS WITH ADHD TO DEVELOP EF SKILLS?

Children with ADHD often lag behind their peers' EF skill development by several years. This EF skills lag is critical for parents to understand in order to have realistic expectations and to offer appropriate EF support. Many parents find themselves struggling to find the right balance, either offering too much external EF support (helicopter parenting), which can prevent their daughter from working on age-appropriate EF skills, or suddenly withdrawing external EF support on critical tasks in later years, which can leave their teen or young adult completely unprepared to make critical life decisions or manage the multiple demands of daily life.

Knowing when and how much to help

Offering external EF support to children and teens is always a difficult balancing act. Often parents can benefit by developing a relationship with a professional who can offer guidance periodically as situations change. Parents should keep in mind that under stress we regress. A teen with ADHD that may be managing fairly well, can suddenly melt down, unable to function in ways that she was capable of earlier, in response to the increased stress of SAT exams, college applications, and increasing expectations from teachers.

Building brain-friendly daily habits

EF skills are also dependent upon a number of factors that relate to general cognitive functioning. For example, EF skills tend to diminish when an individual is sleep-deprived, stressed, frustrated, poorly nourished, hungry, or experiencing cognitive fatigue. We can help girls with ADHD to maximize their EF functioning by minimizing these negative factors as much as possible. (Parents can reference our section on Brain Healthy Daily Habits in Chapter Ten for more information on reducing these factors.)

Have realistic expectations

Girls with ADHD often lag two or more years behind their peers in developing EF skills, and some EF skills may not be strong even in adulthood. While some children are naturally organized and focused, many children need support, structure, and encouragement to learn how to be focused, on-time, organized, and self-controlled as they grow older. Many believe that such expectations tend to be higher for girls. While boys will be boys, girls should be neat and tidy, considerate, and self-controlled. Parents of girls with ADHD need to moderate such expectations and interact in a supportive, encouraging manner.

WHEN PARENTS ARE NOT REALISTIC ABOUT THEIR DAUGHTER'S DEVELOPMENTAL AGE

Many parents feel that consequences are the best teacher. The mother described in the following scene was careful to use appropriate consequences for undesirable behavior. However consequences don't teach a girl with ADHD how to cope with a frustrating situation. Does this scene remind you of interactions at your house?

Scene: Dana, a girl with ADHD, her brother, and parents in a restaurant.

Mom: *Stop kicking against the chair.*
Dana: (pouting) *I'm hungry and there's nothing to do!*
Mom: *You'll just have to be patient.*
Dana: *I'm hungry!*
(Starting to knock her foot against chair.)
Mom: *If you don't stop kicking the chair we're going to have to leave.*
Dana: *Fine, I didn't want to come here anyway!*
Mom: *That's it. We're going to sit in the car while Dad and your brother eat dinner.*

Mom and Dana walk out. Dana is angry and crying.

What has Dana learned in this interaction? Chances are, Dana has learned that she hates to go to this restaurant and that Mom is mean. Mom has unrealistic expectations regarding Dana's ability to tolerate frustration, regulate her emotions, and control restlessness/hyperactivity when she is hungry, tired, and bored. Mom can teach Dana some problem-solving skills by waiting until the current upset is over and then talking to her in a supportive, understanding manner. "Let's think about what would make it better for you next time we go to a restaurant." Mom can make some suggestions and ask Dana for her input too. The following are a few examples.

Problem: Hunger lowers frustration tolerance and emotional control.

Solution: Bring a snack or ask the server for bread and butter as soon as she is seated.

Problem: Restless, impatient behavior is more likely when a girl with ADHD has nothing to occupy her attention and reduce her restlessness.

Solution: Bring a coloring book or storybook for Dana to read, or allow Dana to play a child-appropriate game on Mom's smart phone while waiting for the meal.

By engaging with her child in anticipating problems, Mom is modeling good problem-solving behavior that Dana can gradually learn to do for herself.

HELP YOUR DAUGHTER FIND ISLANDS OF SUCCESS

EF struggles are a daily constant for girls with ADHD. Poor EF performance (being late, forgetful, poorly organized, unprepared) takes a grinding, relentless toll on self-esteem. You can help your daughter in profound ways by helping her to find places, people, or activities in her life where she feels successful and appreciated. One girl with ADHD discovered her special place in a nearby non-profit organization that rescued hurt animals and nursed them back to health. Another found success in a part-time job in a small family business where her employers recognized her capabilities and encouraged her. Yet another found success on the soccer field that served as a positive counter-balance for her academic struggles.

DON'T LET EF STRUGGLES DOMINATE YOUR RELATIONSHIP WITH YOUR DAUGHTER

The most negative aspect of living for a girl with ADHD is the feeling that nothing that she does is right. Don't let your relationship with your daughter focus mainly on what is wrong. She'll try so much harder to develop better EF skills if she feels accepted and encouraged. Work to create a home that provides an oasis for your daughter, a place where she feels good about herself, and a place where EF skills are supported in a constructive, encouraging manner.

PROVIDE ADHD-FRIENDLY SCAFFOLDING TO SUPPORT EMERGING EF SKILLS

Scaffolding, as we have mentioned earlier, refers to supports that can be placed around a girl with ADHD until she masters a new EF skill. Scaffolding can come in many forms — providing company at the kitchen table while she does homework, helping her to get started on a difficult long-term assignment, helping her break big projects into smaller pieces, or hiring a coach or tutor to help support her in areas where she struggles. Scaffolding can be gradually removed as skills are solidified.

CRITICISM TEACHES LOW SELF-ESTEEM, NOT EF SKILLS

So often, adults attempt to teach EF skills through lectures and admonishments. Does the following exchange sound familiar to you?

Ellie: *Mom, I need poster board for my presentation on the environment tomorrow!*
Mom: *I'm not going to the store to buy poster paper now! You should have planned ahead.*
Ellie: (in tears) *Fine! Then I just won't be able to do it and I'll get an F!*
Mom: *Maybe next time you'll remember to plan ahead!*

This mother is trying hard to make her daughter accountable for her actions. The problem is, for a girl with ADHD, this exchange will do little more than make her feel frustrated and angry. Negative consequences don't give her the tools to plan ahead next time. Making Ellie feel bad about her poor planning skills only worsens her self-esteem. Instead, Mom could teach a valuable lesson through a different exchange with Ellie.

Mom: *Ellie, I know you're trying hard to get your work done. So I'd like to help you. But you'll need to help me in return. If I go out to get your poster board, I won't have time to fold the laundry. I'll go get the poster board now if you will fold the laundry while I'm gone.*
Ellie: *Thanks, Mom. I'm sorry I forgot.*
Mom: It's not easy learning to plan ahead. Let's start looking at your assignments on the calendar every day. That way we'll both know what you'll need ahead of time.

In this exchange, Mom is not critical of Ellie, and she's not enabling Ellie to expect her mother to just drop everything when Ellie needs something. She's learning how to make a reasonable exchange — a skill that will serve her well throughout her life.

And because the interaction has been a positive one, Ellie will be more open to her mother's suggestion about developing the habit of planning ahead.

SUPPORT CAN BOTH HELP AND HINDER YOUR DAUGHTER WITH ADHD

The development of EF skills is rarely a smooth path. EF skills tend to falter when stress levels are high. For many girls with ADHD, puberty can feel like an emotional roller coaster. Emotional volatility can take a real toll on emerging EF skills. Again, in high school years, when long-term projects and academic demands increase, more scaffolding may be required while girls learn the skills to organize and manage complex tasks.

Knowing when to provide EF support and when to remove it is one of the critical challenges faced by parents as they guide their child toward adult independence. Too much support deprives your daughter from taking the reins and developing confidence that she can learn to take charge of her own life. Too little support and your daughter may become so discouraged that she underestimates her potential, lowering her goals in order to lower her stress.

SOME EF SKILLS MAY ALWAYS PROVE CHALLENGING FOR YOUR DAUGHTER

One of the critical skills needed to live well with ADHD is an understanding of what sorts of tasks will always require support, and what sorts of tasks should probably be outsourced, even in adulthood. In addition to developing EF skills, girls with ADHD need to grow into women who understand their strengths and limitations. They will need to learn how to find appropriate support throughout their lives. Support can come from a spouse, roommate, friends, relatives, ADHD support groups, ADHD coaches, and professional organizers. So help your daughter to understand that no one is good at everything, and that the smart course is to look for help when you need it, before a situation has become critical.

A SHORT LIST OF WAYS TO HELP YOUR DAUGHTER BUILD STRONGER EF SKILLS

Build working memory

Working memory is memory for things that we need to keep in short term memory for our immediate use. For example, we use our working memory to recall multistep instructions. You may have noticed that your daughter has difficulty remembering when you ask her to do more than one thing at the same time.

- To help your daughter, make it into a game in which she challenges herself and keeps track of how many things she can recall correctly.

- Give her multistep directions, and then ask her to repeat them back before she follows them.

- Games such as *grocery store,* in which two children keep adding grocery store items to a growing list which they must recall and then add to, is a game that calls for working memory.

- Help her to learn strategies, such as writing the steps down, if she is unable to keep them in her working memory.

Increase persistence

Make it into a game with your daughter. Rather than chiding her when she quits a task, challenge her to persevere until a specific point and then reward and praise her for her growing perseverance.

For example:

- Ask her to read increasing numbers of pages of assigned reading. If she gets tired and frustrated after two to three pages, challenge her to see if she can persist until she has read four pages. Gradually increase the task as she consistently succeeds at the current level.

- Tell her about *The Little Engine That Could* – a story that highlights persistence in the face of a difficult task. Then make it into a game to become the *Little Engine* as she tackles daunting tasks, such as picking up a large number of toys or personal items.

Learn to get started

Many girls with ADHD experience difficulty getting started on a task. To help your daughter learn to get started on her own, talk about initiation as a specific kind of task that requires specific techniques.

Barriers to getting started:

1. Lack of materials — help your daughter make a list of necessary materials.

2. Lack of appropriate space to do the task — help her to choose an appropriate uncluttered space in which to work on the task.

3. The task feels too large — help her to break the task into tiny bites — then get started by completing the first bite. A bite can be something that takes as little as 10 minutes.

4. Involvement in a more appealing activity — teach your daughter to earn appealing activities by completing bites of her long-term project.

Improve time awareness

For people with ADHD, time often feels very elastic and difficult to track. Some tools that can assist your daughter in learning to keep track of time:

1. Audible timers — these timers can be set to call out the number of minutes left — "Nine minutes" — and can be very helpful in keeping your daughter on track as she is in preparation to leave for school or for some other activity that requires a specific departure time. They are also a good way to track time until bedtime.

2. Time Timer*tm* —The Time Timer*tm* is a timer that presents a bold visual representation of how much time is remaining. The maximum time that can be set is one hour. The remaining time is shown in bright red – so if you set the Time Timer*tm* for one hour, the full clock face is red and gradually reduces as the clock face turns counter-clockwise. Glancing at a Time Timer*tm* can give your daughter a quick visual report on time remaining, helping her to keep her efforts on track.

3. Calendars — are important to help your daughter become more aware of time over longer ranges.

4. Agendas — by middle school, your daughter should be learning to use a daily agenda to list each day's events and tasks. Do this with her in a brief daily planning session – 5-10 minutes in the evening to plan the next day.

Reduce forgetfulness

Forgetfulness is a pattern that your daughter may need to work against throughout her life. Several tools to lessen forgetfulness are:

1. Developing routines — morning routines, house departure routines, home arrival routines, homework routines, and bedtime routines. Routines reduce forgetfulness because they are a sequence of tasks or actions that are repeated over and over in the same order. Once a routine has become habitual, few reminders should be necessary. Creating an easy-to-read poster board listing the steps of each routine, in order, is very helpful to children (and adults) in building a routine.

2. Setting alarms — an easy tool to remind a child of a future action or task is to set an audible reminder. As your daughter becomes used to using an audible reminder system, the responsibility for setting the alarm should gradually shift from parent to child.

3. Creative reminders — the same reminders won't work for everyone, but working together with your daughter, you can gradually develop reminders that work for her. Make a list of things that she frequently forgets, then problem-solve with her to develop reminders that work. If the first reminder you decide upon doesn't seem to be effective, go back to problem-solving until you find one that works.

Improve planning skills

Planning skills are best introduced in planning activities that are pleasurable for your daughter. Once she has developed some planning skills, then it's much easier for her to apply them to activities that may be more difficult or less pleasant – such as working on a challenging school assignment. Cooking a favorite dessert together is a great way to help a girl learn to plan. Lots of steps are involved, and the end of the project is sweet success. Girls can learn to plan by participating in the planning of a birthday party, a week-end outing, or an art project at home. When we teach planning skills through enjoyable activities, a girl with ADHD learns a very immediate lesson about how learning to plan leads to achieving what she wants.

Organization of things

Keeping things organized when you are a girl with ADHD is very daunting. You can help your daughter learn to become better organized by teaching her a few key ideas:

1. Downsize your daughter's belongings. Your daughter may feel very attached to outgrown clothing, favorite books or toys that she no longer uses, or papers and mementos. Instead of expecting her to get rid of things that she's attached to, help her to downsize to things that she uses frequently at the moment. It's easy enough to pack up outgrown clothing, toys, and books and store them in the attic, basement, garage or storage unit.

2. A place for everything. Make storage containers clearly assigned and easily accessible. Labels are great reminders of where things live. The easier the access, the more likely the storage containers will be used.

3. Tie the bow! Tying the bow is the last step when you are wrapping up a package — so teach your daughter to tie the bow on each activity she engages in. Most of life's clutter consists of incomplete actions — the coat that was taken off, but not hung up; the materials that were used for a school project that weren't put away. Tying the bow is much easier when there is a clear place where each of her belongings lives.

These are just a few ideas of how parents can help their daughters with ADHD begin to build strong executive functioning skills. Remember, brain development is on your side. The older your daughter grows and the more mature her prefrontal lobes become, the easier it will be for her to demonstrate good EF skills.

CHAPTER NINE

Helping Girls with ADHD Function Well in School

MANY OF OUR DAUGHTERS WITH ADHD face multiple challenges in their efforts to receive the educational supports that they need. Let's look at some of the reasons why girls with ADHD are so often overlooked in school.

First, most girls have not been trained to be assertive, and girls whose self-esteem has been damaged are even less prepared to ask for what they need. Girls with ADHD also create fewer difficulties for the classroom teacher. Most teachers will, quite naturally, focus on those students (more often boys with ADHD) who are causing problems in the classroom.

In addition, the demand for special services greatly exceeds the supply, and girls with ADHD are unlikely to be at the head of the line.

Despite these many obstacles, there is hopeful news as well. Understanding and identification of girls with ADHD has greatly improved in recent years. ADHD research involving girls has increased and a picture of the significance of coexisting conditions has emerged, allowing for a clearer delineation of the needs of girls with ADHD and the development of specialized programs to increase opportunities for success.

In this chapter, we will introduce a range of approaches that have been demonstrated to help girls with ADHD in school. Parents are encouraged to create a team of individuals, both within and outside of the school, that work together to help their daughter with ADHD to recognize and realize her full potential. This team might consist of teachers, counselors and school psychologists, as well as outside service providers, such as psychologists, tutors, ADHD coaches, occupational therapists, and physicians, if medication is part of the girl's treatment regimen. Certainly not all girls with ADHD need all of these interventions. To whatever extent possible, parents should seek available supports and services within the school setting in order to manage the cost of necessary educational supports.

VOICES FROM THE PAST
GROWING UP WITHOUT DIAGNOSIS, ACCOMMODATIONS, OR SUPPORT

Before we begin to outline educational approaches that can better support our daughters with ADHD, let's listen to the voices of women who did not have the benefit of identification and support during their school years. Perhaps by hearing their accounts we can develop a clearer notion of how to respond to the needs of girls growing up today.

Sally, now in her forties, was a bright, athletic tomboy who grew up climbing trees and competing with her brothers. Although very outgoing, Sally recalls preferring the company of boys, with whom she felt more at home, to the company of her female peers, where she never quite fit in.

> *"When I was in school teachers would say that I never stopped talking. I was very social; always busy doing something, and not paying attention to my lessons. On my report cards only one teacher caught it (her ADHD) and said that I was inconsistent and made careless errors. The other teachers just patted me on the head and said I was fine.*
>
> *No one expected me to be a scholar. I was told my whole life that I was average. I didn't make A's and no one expected me to. I earned a strong B average with no effort. I didn't realize I was smart until I got to college, but even there I had no direction and kept changing my major every time I met a professor that I liked.*
>
> *With more guidance and structure I would have been able to develop, but, as it was, it felt like I was slogging through a swamp, trying to get where I was going, but every step I sank down to my knees. I kept going, but I never knew where I was."*

Sally's experience is a common one for bright, active girls with ADHD. She functioned well enough to get along on the strength of her native ability, but spent many wasted years, underestimating her ability and having no clear sense of direction. Looking back, Sally believes that more guidance and structure would have been of great benefit, but teachers and parents didn't expect much of her. It was only much later that she came to have higher expectations for herself.

Mary (portions of her poem in Chapter One are included here) had a very different self-image than Sally. While Sally was physically active and competitive, the tomboy variety of ADHD in girls, Mary was quiet, artistic and non-assertive. She had very little success in school and grew up believing herself to be dumb. In her forties, Mary was diagnosed with ADHD, and only then was able to acknowledge her artistic ability. Mary worked hard to come to terms with who she is and to overcome the very low self-esteem from which she suffered during her school years.

School overwhelmed me
I couldn't understand
Just how to behave
To fit into their plan.

The classes were long,
I could not stay clear.
My brain was so busy
Pretending to hear.

I dreaded the clock
And its torturous pace.
I could never keep up,
I would just lose my place.

For years I felt less than
With no self-esteem.
I thought I was stupid
Began to careen . . .

As Mary's poem continues, she describes her descent, during high school years, into promiscuity, desperately seeking a positive response from boys — the only arena where she experienced success.

Anne-Marie, like Mary, was also on the quiet, non-hyperactive side of the ADHD equation, but presented a more complex and puzzling picture because she was able to excel, academically, in some areas. At the same time, however, Anne-Marie had enormous difficulty concentrating while reading. As a result, she rarely read for pleasure. She was so clearly capable and talented in music and writing that her reading difficulties were dismissed as laziness.

"I was a quiet kid. No one really noticed me at school, apart from the ones that enjoyed reading my stories or my flute playing. I had trouble socializing with the other kids and stuck to one friend who was trustworthy. I was quiet, but sometimes, when I did open my mouth, I said the wrong thing.

School days were hell. I was bullied and didn't know how to stick up for myself. I could never find the right words. Although I was praised for my English essays, I struggled with reading comprehension. I loved stories, but I avoided books as I found it difficult to concentrate. My dad would often accuse me of being lazy because I didn't read.

All through school I felt ugly and stupid. However, I got through it because I thought I would grow out of it. I would constantly fantasize about the person I was going to be. Anne-Marie, the famous musician. Anne-Marie the record producer. But, it seems I never did grow up. Now, at 29, I'm still that insecure, highly emotional, scatty little girl who daydreams all the time."

Anne-Marie had big dreams, but mostly they were daydreams, with no concrete plan to implement them. She comforted herself with daydreams while she suffered from teasing, criticism and highly variable grades. As a young adult, she remained stuck, drifting, and full of self-recrimination.

Three different stories: Sally, the athletic tomboy, and Mary, the shy, quiet girl whose abilities were greatly underestimated; and Anne Marie, clearly talented in music and writing, but written off by her teachers as lazy when her overall academic record did not match her recognized ability.

"Sweet, but not very bright; talented but lazy; an average girl who is doing just fine." Different explanations, but all three are classic ways that girls with ADHD are diminished and gradually learn to discount themselves and their abilities.

WHY HAVE GIRLS BEEN OVERLOOKED IN THE CLASSROOM?

Socialization patterns for girls

Thom Hartmann, a widely read author on ADHD, and father of a daughter with ADHD, writes that one of the major reasons that girls are overlooked in schools has to do with the way that parents, with or without awareness, train their sons and daughters differently.

"In our culture we tell two stories, no matter how enlightened we may be. Little boys are told that if they have a need they should meet it in the environment. Boys are taught to acquire physical, interpersonal power, but little girls are told to internalize — "Sit down, be quiet, be a lady." Boys learn to reach out and grab when they need stimulation; girls learn how to achieve stimulation inside their own heads." [1]

Whether we attribute the behavior of most girls that place them in the primarily inattentive type ADHD to the socialization process that Thom Hartmann describes, or to inborn physiological, temperamental differences, our task remains the same — to empower girls with ADHD to ask for what they need and to teach them that they are in school to learn and grow, not just to please the teacher and stay out of trouble.

Teacher ADHD questionnaires are not designed to identify the internalized struggles of most girls with ADHD. As Thom Hartmann[2] described, for many girls with ADHD their disorder is an internalized one. While boys with ADHD may externalize their needs — through demanding, arguing, fighting, resisting or disrupting, many girls do not manifest their needs and feelings externally. One of the best ways to find out about a girl's needs is to ask — in a setting where a girl can feel safe and secure. For girls age 10 and above, a self-report form may prove very beneficial, if the teacher notes any of the behavior patterns listed above, suggestive of ADHD. For girls under the age of 10, a verbal interview with the girl and her parent or parents may yield better information. A teacher should keep in mind that many girls won't *show* you, but, if they feel safe, they might *tell* you what is wrong. A Self-report Scale to help uncover the internal struggles of these girls with ADHD may be found in the appendix on page 305.

GIRLS TRY HARDER! AT GREAT COST TO THEMSELVES

Before girls with ADHD can be helped, they must first be identified – not always an easy process. Just as a chameleon strives to hide, to blend in with its surroundings, to camouflage itself, so do many girls with ADHD attempt a disappearing act in the classroom. It's no wonder that teachers often overlook them. They can be hard to spot — partly because many of them do not fit the standard ADHD profile that teachers have been taught to recognize, and also because many girls go to great effort to escape their teacher's notice.

Girls with ADHD may easily go unnoticed because they intensely over-function, fueled by anxiety-driven efforts to please teachers and parents. Young women commonly report that "my teachers never knew how hard I worked to earn the grades I received." Parents, however, are all too familiar with their daughter's effort and anxiety because they are there to observe their daughter's meltdowns and pattern of working late into the night to complete an assignment or prepare for an exam. As is true of girls in general,[3] girls with ADHD demonstrate better self-control and fewer oppositional behaviors toward the teacher.[4]

While academic functioning is important, girls who work incredibly hard to keep up with academic demands can still suffer significant damage to their self-esteem, identity development, and social functioning while earning good grades. "What's wrong with me?" many of these girls ask, "Why do I have to work so much harder than everyone else?" And, to add insult to injury, sometimes their painfully earned grades are used as evidence that they have no need of academic support.

In viewing the academic progression of girls with ADHD, it is easy to forget the extreme effort often required of them to achieve these goals. The fact that they make these extreme efforts, often involving chronic anxiety, desperate all-night efforts, feelings of being overwhelmed, struggling as they try to write papers and complete projects, should not be used as evidence that they need no accommodations or assistance.

TEACHERS ARE MORE FAMILIAR WITH BOYS' ADHD BEHAVIORS

Often, lack of knowledge and recognition on the part of teachers and parents lead us to overlook many girls with ADHD. Because the current guidelines better describe boys than girls with ADHD, teachers may know that something is amiss, but won't interpret a girl's difficulties as signs of ADHD. The result is that many girls do not receive badly needed support and educational interventions.

HIGH IQ GIRLS CAN FUNCTION WELL DESPITE ADHD FOR MANY YEARS

Girls with high IQ and ADHD are often not identified as being either gifted or ADHD. Their executive functioning challenges can mask their ability, while their ability allows them to maintain grades that can readily mask ADHD. Bright women with ADHD, diagnosed as adults, report that their high potential was unrecognized, and their grade-level performance was viewed as adequate. They received no assistance with executive functioning, and, what's worse, their average grade-level performance was seen as all that they were capable of achieving.

Some mental health professionals, even today, mistakenly believe that one cannot succeed academically and yet have ADHD. While evidence of some signs of ADHD should be present from early childhood, bright children with ADHD, especially females, may be found among the top students in the early grades. One study examined gifted students and found that a subgroup of them qualified for an ADHD diagnosis despite very strong cognitive abilities. Gifted students with ADHD differed from their non-ADHD peers in a number of ways. They had more close family members diagnosed with ADHD and demonstrated more associated psychopathology including anxiety, depression, and PTSD (post-traumatic stress disorder), among others.[5]

Often, in high school, ADHD patterns become more evident as academic demands increase. However, it is quite possible to graduate from college and even earn an advanced degree, and yet have ADHD. Sadly, however, many bright people fall along the wayside, never completing their advanced degree, due to lack of diagnosis and treatment. While supporting research remains to be done, it seems likely that ADHD is overrepresented among doctoral degree candidates who have never completed their degree, as well as among students who have difficulty passing their medical board exams or bar exams. Yet, regrettably, many parents are told that their high IQ daughter's grade-level work renders her ineligible for supports or accommodations along the way.

HELPING CLASSROOM TEACHERS TO RECOGNIZE AND IDENTIFY ADHD IN GIRLS

> *I would be too embarrassed to raise my hand, fearing that I would look dumb. And sometimes I didn't even know how to*

put my thoughts into words to ask what I didn't understand!

Teachers can find girls' ADHD parent-report questionnaires at the end of each school-age-related chapter (elementary through high school), while a general girls self-report questionnaire can be found at the end of this book. Teachers are encouraged to use these questionnaires as screening devices. While they are not formal, normed diagnostic tools, they can be used very effectively as an initial screening. If a girl responds positively to a majority of the items, it may be appropriate to communicate to the parents that a full evaluation may be warranted.

To begin to identify girls who may need to be assessed for ADHD, teachers should be on the look-out for girls who:

- talk compulsively.
- look attentive, but when called upon are often not able to answer a question.
- have difficulty following directions.
- frequently ask other students to repeat the teacher's instructions.
- sit quietly, appearing to work, but rarely finish their assignments.
- have desks or lockers that are much messier than those of their classmates.
- often forget to turn in permission slips.
- forget to turn in homework that has been completed.
- frequently don't have all of the supplies they need in class.
- seem to have auditory processing problems.
- seem to have expressive language problems.
- tend to work very slowly.

OTHER LEARNING DIFFERENCES NEED TO BE RECOGNIZED AND ADDRESSED

It's almost never *just* ADHD. As we discussed elsewhere in this book, ADHD is a condition that usually is accompanied by one or more associated disorders. In the school setting, all traits and areas of relative academic weakness need to be addressed in order to help a girl with ADHD function up to her potential. Reading disorders (RD) and ADHD are very often found together.[6] Inattentive girls, in particular, have been found to be much more prone to reading disorders than girls with combined type ADHD.[7] Disorders of written expression are five times more likely in students with ADHD, and girls with ADHD that also have a reading disorder are even more likely than their male counterparts to have a written language disorder. [8]

One study [9] found that children with ADHD that were without reading disabilities nevertheless were inefficient verbal learners. Students with ADHD recalled less than their non-ADHD peers, although girls with ADHD outperformed boys with ADHD and demonstrated stronger learning strategies. The implications of this study are that girls with ADHD will have more difficulty listening and recalling names, dates and terminology and will require more time and repetition in order to master the information.

PARENTS' ADVOCACY ROLE

Parents who suspect that their daughter may have attentional problems should not rely solely upon the classroom teacher to make this identification. If the teacher or school does not recognize attentional difficulties in their daughter, they should seek a private evaluation from a professional who has experience in working with girls, and who recognizes the diverse histories and patterns that girls with ADHD may demonstrate. Following a private diagnosis, they can then approach the school, asking for a teacher conference to discuss the findings and to request specific accommodations.

Parents need to educate themselves as much as possible about ADHD, especially about ADHD in girls. They may have to play a strong advocacy and education role within the educational system in order to make their daughter's needs clear and to obtain the services and supports that will help her achieve to her potential. The good news is that teacher awareness and education about girls with ADHD has improved in recent years, making it more likely that the school will actively partner with parents in securing these necessary supports and accommodations.

PARENTAL ADVOCACY CANNOT ADDRESS ALL NEEDS OF GIRLS WITH ADHD

Because girls with ADHD often present differently than boys with the disorder, and have more internalizing symptoms such as anxiety and depression, sometimes even ardent advocacy is not enough to gain the needed supports and accommodations.

> *The modern classroom has proven basically toxic for Mindy. The exciting, noisy, visually stimulating, socially intense classroom we have today just overwhelms her. She is strong academically, yet performs inconsistently. Third grade has been catastrophic for her. A myriad of well-intentioned professionals can't fathom how someone can be very bright and very good in academic tasks and still*

> *have learning and attention differences severe enough to impair functioning. They also can't understand the toll taken even by successful coping mechanisms.*

The comments of Mindy's mother reveal the great and typically hidden cost of coping mechanisms utilized by girls with ADHD. Out of an internal pressure to please, girls are more prone to struggle to do what is expected of them, to make enormous efforts, for which they are sometimes punished through denial of accommodations. A girl's level of effort and degree of anxiety must be taken into account, not just her ability to meet grade level expectations.

> *This year, even when Mindy had a diagnosis of ADHD, had been taking Ritalin for over a year, was receiving informal accommodations, and was making daily visits to the clinic (just to get out of the stressful class), the local screening committee decided she was ineligible for a 504 plan because she was at or above grade level in all her academic subjects.*

Mindy's mother goes on to relate that her daughter's stress level led to increasing depression and anxiety. As expectations escalated, Mindy reacted with panic, on occasion refusing to attend school. Ultimately, the school responded, not with a 504 plan, but with placement in a class for the emotionally disturbed. Mindy was very unhappy in this class, and exhibited increasing depression. Ironically, her depression was interpreted as evidence that this class for the emotionally disturbed was the appropriate placement for her. Her parents and psychiatrist strongly disagreed because they saw the other Mindy — the creative, compassionate, kind, strong, incredibly intelligent, incredibly lonely Mindy. They believed that her school placement was highly destructive for her and have searched far and wide for alternatives instead of returning her to the program for the emotionally disturbed following her summer break. Both Mindy's mother and her psychiatrist strongly believed that her anxiety and depression were secondary to her ADHD, and that what she needed were the structures and supports appropriate for a gifted child with ADHD.

Mindy's troubling, even tragic story is an extreme example of the types of difficulties that can be experienced by girls with ADHD — who are more likely to be compliant, anxious, overwhelmed, and depressed. Inadequate supports for a very sensitive, gifted girl with ADHD have created a situation in which her secondary emotional reaction is now seen as her primary diagnosis!

WHAT DO GIRLS WITH ADHD NEED FROM THEIR SCHOOLS?

In early childhood, executive functioning (EF) skills, more than IQ, are predictors of reading and math skills throughout the school years.[10, 11] As educators are increasingly aware of the link between strong executive functioning abilities to academic achievement, increasing attention has been focused on how to improve a student's EF skills. In this section we will briefly touch on a range of evidence-based interventions that can be undertaken in the school setting.

Working in small group settings

It is important to understand that the learning context is also key for students with ADHD. It has been reported that students with ADHD demonstrate significant improvement in focus and on-task behavior when they work in small groups. These same students show much less focus and on-task behavior when either working alone or working on a classroom-wide level.[12] These findings need to be kept in mind when selecting a teaching strategy for girls with ADHD.

Mindfulness training in the classroom

Mindfulness training has been used in the classroom with children as young as age six or seven with very positive gains in executive functioning skills. Mindfulness training in the classroom has involved a sitting meditation to increase attentional awareness as well as walking mindfulness exercises such as walking a line carefully while holding a spoon filled with water. Teachers and parents have both reported increased executive functioning skills as mindfulness training continues.[13]

Teaching emotional control and problem-solving skills

The PATHS Program (Promoting Alternative-Thinking Strategies) is a teacher led program to help children learn to respond to problems or upset by:

1. stopping,
2. taking a deep breath,
3. verbalizing their feelings,
4. practicing conscious self-control over emotional reactions, and
5. developing a plan of action to address the problem.

Teachers are encouraged to have students use this approach in different situations throughout the school day. Studies have shown a significant increase in self-control and planful problem-solving in children exposed to this program.[14, 15]

Computer training to improve attention and working memory

Several computer training programs have been developed to

improve executive functioning skills. One of the best known is Cogmed™ designed to improve working memory. Research suggests that such programs are only helpful if the programs are used very consistently and at increasing levels of difficulty. It is not clear how much the improvement in working memory skills transfers to other working memory tasks within the academic setting.[16]

Directed attention

Research has shown that children with ADHD can improve their skills in working math problems when key words in the math problems are highlighted for them, drawing their attention to elements necessary to solve the problem. There is evidence that after practicing word problems with highlighting, these skills transfer to non-highlighted word problems, suggesting that this type of cueing aids students in learning to attend to salient words or cues.[17]

Instruction in setting and meeting goals

Many students with ADHD set goals to avoid feelings of shame or inadequacy — in other words, their goal is to avoid performance in order to avoid demonstrating their inadequacy.[18] Moving students from a goal-avoidant pattern to a goal-achieving pattern requires careful, consistent structuring on the part of the teacher. Goals should be clearly defined, should have a very short-term deadline (in ½ hour; today; tonight), and should be a small enough incremental increase in demand that the student has a high probability of success – clear, soon, and do-able. Success breeds success. Small incremental improvements, defined as success, will help build confidence that will motivate the student toward meeting the next goal.

Introduce and practice daily various organizational strategies

Organizing strategies, such as creating a checklist for segments of a writing assignment or using a calendar system to schedule tasks do not come easily to students with ADHD. Even adults with ADHD experience difficulty in consistently using a tool or organizing strategy. Teachers (and parents) need to structure and support practice sessions on a daily basis until the use of these organizing tools becomes second nature to the girl with ADHD.

HOW CAN TEACHERS CREATE AN ADHD-FRIENDLY CLASSROOM FOR GIRLS?

What's good for ADHD is good for everyone. Instead of attempting the impossible task of following detailed 504 Plans or IEPs (two different types of plans for the educational accommodation of students with a disability or medical condition that impacts learning), why not create a classroom that accommodates differences and supports needs of all students? Below are some ways to create a more ADHD-friendly classroom setting.

Provide frequent encouragement

One issue that girls with ADHD consistently describe, whether they fall on the hyperactive/hypersocial side or on the quiet, daydreamy side of the ADHD spectrum, is a sense of embarrassment or shame in the classroom. Some may deal with this feeling by showing an attitude of resentment ("The best defense is a good offense."); others by clowning and joking ("If I'm silly and entertaining, no one will notice that I never know what page we're on."); by ingratiating themselves to their teacher ("If she likes me, then maybe she won't get mad at me."); and still others by attempting to disappear ("If I hide, then I won't get in trouble.") Due to low self-esteem, self-blame, and feelings of shame, what almost none of them do is to express their fears and embarrassment to their teacher. Without adequate explanation, the teacher is left to her own devices to understand why Sally is frequently absent from school, is never finished with her desk work, or is usually jabbering to the kid sitting next to her.

Assign her a study buddy

Rather than admonishing a girl for not listening to directions, the ADHD-sensitive teacher can give her explicit permission to quietly ask her study buddy what to do. The shy, withdrawn, insecure girl with ADHD may be best placed next to a well-organized, friendly student from whom she can ask assistance without embarrassment. Studies have demonstrated that feelings of loneliness and isolation negatively impact EF skills.[19] A study buddy is a readily available cost-free intervention.

Provide peer tutoring

Allow students that have thoroughly mastered a topic to help other students that are still struggling. This accommodates the student in need of more one-on-one attention as well as the student that may be gifted and bored and requires more stimulation.

Approach her with warmth and encouragement

A teacher can explicitly encourage these girls to come to him or her for extra support, and can more frequently cruise by her desk to redirect and encourage her. Girls with ADHD tend to respond much better to praise and encouragement than to criticism and negative consequences.

Make the classroom feel safe

In the most general sense, the teacher can give great support to a girl with ADHD through making the classroom a comfort zone — where she can feel safe to make mistakes, to ask the teacher to repeat herself, or to explain that, yet again, she has forgotten to bring in her homework.

Allow frequent movement breaks

Recognize that a girl with ADHD may need more frequent movement breaks than her fellow students.

Collaboratively problem-solve with her

Rather than criticize her for losing or forgetting something, engage her in collaborative problem-solving, while recognizing that such lapses will occur occasionally, despite the best laid plans.

Avoid calling on the shy, inattentive girl

Make a pact with her that she will be called upon only when she raises her hand, indicating that she knows the answer.

Encourage her to come to the teacher's desk

A private conversation to offer an explanation if she's feeling confused or unsure of how to proceed will support her without embarrassing her in front of her peers.

Maximize praise, minimize criticism

The more her teacher can recognize a girl with ADHD for her curiosity, creativity, and enthusiasm, while de-emphasizing her forgetfulness, inattention, or disorganization, the young female student with ADHD can develop the building blocks of self-esteem which will help her develop into a confident young woman who believes in her own capabilities.

ELEMENTARY SCHOOL ACCOMMODATIONS FOR ADHD TO MINIMIZE ITS IMPACT

- Seat the compulsive talker away from her best friends, letting her know that this is not meant as a punishment, but as a way to support her in getting her work done.
- Minimize the need to transport papers to and from school. Allow her to email her assignments from home.
- Use the internet — to post homework assignments, list questions or problems for test review, and information for parents.
- Reduce the number of questions or assigned problems for students with slow processing speed. Many students can adequately learn and can demonstrate that learning without completing as many items as have been assigned to the whole class.
- Suggest to parents that they purchase voice-to-text software that allows a student to dictate a paper or book report.
- Allow retaking of tests to accommodate the inconsistency of ADHD performance. The goal of education is to learn and to be able to demonstrate that learning, not to pass or fail a test on a particular day.
- Provide oral exams for girls with ADHD whose verbal expressive skills far surpass their written language skills.
- Don't mark off for messiness. While this may be a sign of decreased effort for students without ADHD, poor handwriting, erasures, and general messiness are hallmarks of ADHD written work. The most constructive solution is the early development of keyboarding skills. It's much easier to push a key than to copy a letter of the alphabet, and erasures

on the computer screen are invisible, allowing the student with ADHD to eventually produce a neat, legible product.

- Give students with ADHD stronger encouragement to develop keyboarding skills by making daily keyboarding practice a routine for them in the classroom. Fifteen minutes a day with a keyboarding program can help a child to rapidly progress in keyboarding skills.
- Recognize that daydreaming is often beyond her control. Draw her back to attention discretely, without teasing or criticizing.
- Lecture for shorter periods of time and engage all of your students, ADHD or not, through more class discussion and interaction.
- Recognize that transitions can be difficult for her. She may have become so involved in one activity that she doesn't hear you tell the class that it's time for another subject.
- Recognize that a very bright child can also leave her backpack in the aisle without it being a sign of inconsiderateness.
- Accommodate memory retrieval problems. It has been found that students with ADHD had difficulty retrieving information that they had demonstrably learned earlier.[20] Because information retrieval is so inconsistent in students with ADHD, tests should be modified to allow them to demonstrate what they *can* recall rather than catching them on what they learned but can't recall. Test questions with more open-ended answers or verbal administration of a test that allows the teacher to explore the student's actual level of content mastery can at least partially accommodate the faulty retrieval system of a student with ADHD.

ACCOMMODATIONS FOR GIRLS WITH ADHD IN THE UPPER GRADES

As girls move from elementary to middle and high school, challenges increase and life becomes increasingly complex. The need for accommodations and services is typically much greater during these years. Girls move from a single teacher to multiple teachers, and homework assignments and reading requirements lengthen. Executive functioning challenges take a greater toll as demands for organization and long-term planning greatly increase. Social pressures increase and become more complex as boy/girl relationships come into the picture, social cliques form, and one's identity is increasingly dependent upon social groups and extracurricular activities.

In adolescence, expectations rise that girls should generally be able to function more independent of structure and guidance provided by parents and teachers. Meanwhile, hormonal changes and fluctuations tend to increase mood lability and to intensify the impact of ADHD patterns.

CLASSROOM/TEACHER ACCOMMODATIONS APPROPRIATE IN UPPER GRADES

- A note-taker (or access to the teacher's notes) for class lectures so that the student can listen and interact without needing to simultaneously take detailed notes.

- Extended time on tests.
- Provision of a separate, quiet room in which to take tests.
- Alternative forms of tests, including essay tests and oral examinations.
- Reasonable flexibility in meeting deadlines.
- Extra text books available in the classroom for times when the text may have been accidentally left at home or in the locker.
- Internet posting of homework assignments, guidelines for long-term assignments, and dates of upcoming quizzes, tests, and due dates of papers and projects.
- Allowing students to turn in homework via email, thus reducing the possibility that students can misplace or forget to turn in assignments.

(It is important for high school teachers to be aware that all of these accommodations, aside from extra textbooks, are typically available on the college campus, and are needed even more on the high school level.)

CREATING AN ADHD-FRIENDLY SCHOOL
SCHOOL-WIDE SUPPORTS FOR GIRLS WITH ADHD

What kind of supports should the school offer as girls move from the classroom cocoon of elementary school to the relative independence of middle and high school?

Need for support that may be ongoing into adulthood

Many teachers feel that it is their mandate, when working with adolescent students, to prepare them for independent living after high school. They repeatedly give students messages about the real world after high school, admonishing them that there will be no one to remind them, to organize them or to guide them, and that they need to practice and prepare for this imminent state of independence. What these teachers often don't realize is that students with ADHD will continue to struggle with problems of forgetfulness, distractibility, and disorganization throughout their lives. The goal of independent living, without supports, in adulthood is neither necessary nor realistic for all adults with ADHD. In fact, feeling the pressure to achieve these goals often triggers feelings of demoralization or hopelessness. An important aspect of success as an adult with ADHD is learning how to find and surround oneself with the supports necessary to function well. High school is the place to begin to identify and put these types of support into place. These students will need organizational supports in high school, in college, and in the workplace as adults, as well as in their personal lives. The challenge for middle and high school teachers is to provide structure and support for students with ADHD, while encouraging them to develop independence in areas in which they are capable.

Provide an ADHD counselor/coach

As students with ADHD move from a single teacher in elementary school, to multiple teachers in middle and high school, they will greatly benefit from having one person with whom they can check in on a frequent basis. This advisor/coach/counselor can help them learn to schedule, prioritize, and organize the multiple demands from multiple teachers. While the need for such coaching and study skills training has been recognized and provided for some time on the college level, most middle and high schools do not yet offer the services of such a support person.

Offer school-based support groups

Girls with ADHD, much more frequently than boys with ADHD, report feeling socially isolated, different from their peers, and very unhappy in this isolation. While support programs focus more on academic support, and on methods to control rebellious or antagonistic behavior during adolescence, little attention has been paid to the social anxieties that are of such great concern for girls with ADHD. Importantly, loneliness has been demonstrated to decrease executive functioning skills.[21] Support groups can provide a safe place where a girl with ADHD feels that she belongs and is accepted.

The best way that we can help inoculate these girls against these risks is to help them to develop interests and talents, to help them feel a sense of commonality with other girls struggling with similar issues, and to give them positive role models. A girls' support group, headed by a school counselor or psychologist is an ideal way to provide such support.

Priority, customized registration

Rising at an early hour to concentrate in seven different classes during a long, tiring, and distracting day is a challenge for all adolescents, but often poses an all but impossible challenge for teens with ADHD. One of the most important ways that schools can accommodate the teen with ADHD is to customize her registration so that her most challenging classes are taught at optimal times of day, with less challenging classes interspersed among those that are most challenging for her. If she is provided with an ADHD counselor or coach at the middle and high school level, someone who knows her strengths and weaknesses, this is the ideal person to help her arrange for customized registration at the beginning of each term. Colleges and universities very commonly provide this accommodation to students with ADHD, however very few middle and high schools have instituted similar policies.

Self-advocacy training

All students with ADHD need to make the successful transition to advocating for their own educational needs from a dependency upon their parents, who typically play this role through their early school years. Girls with ADHD have a special need to learn self-advocacy because of their ADHD tendency to hide, to be self-effacing, and to feel too embarrassed or threatened to make their needs known. Girls that have hidden for years in elementary school, depending upon their mother to talk to their teachers and counselors, have a long journey to reach the point where they can successfully advocate for themselves, especially as they encounter skeptical or non-supportive teachers in high school and beyond.

Unfortunately, many high school counselors emphasize the need for self-advocacy without providing any training to make it possible. And girls, who have been taught since earliest childhood, to accommodate, to adapt, to internalize have a much greater challenge than their male counterparts in learning to speak up for themselves. A girls' ADHD support group could also provide an excellent setting in which to develop these advocacy skills.

Introduce a school-wide aerobic exercise program

Several studies have shown a very strong increase in executive functioning following aerobic exercise. Aerobic exercise specifically, rather than physical education in general, shows much stronger EF benefits.[22] Several schools have experimentally included universal mandatory aerobic exercise in their curriculum to very positive effect.[23]

ALTERNATIVES TO PUBLIC SCHOOL

Private schools

One alternative to public schools, albeit an expensive one, is to find a private school setting which is more appropriate to the needs of the girl with ADHD. Because girls with ADHD are diverse, the ideal academic setting for one girl may actually be inappropriate for another. Parents, whose budgets allow, may benefit from seeking the assistance of a school placement specialist in selecting a school. Some girls with ADHD, especially those of the shy, inattentive type, may thrive in a school that offers small class size and a very personalized, supportive teaching style. Others may thrive in a highly structured school setting that offers supervised study periods and structured help in learning to plan and to organize. Yet some girls may find such a setting too controlling and confining, and may thrive in a school that emphasizes creativity and independence. A few very bright girls with ADHD may not qualify for gifted programs within the public school system due to mediocre grades. However, a private school that recognizes their talents and can challenge them academically may allow a girl with high IQ to feel more stimulated and motivated. Some private schools are in a better position to individualize the teaching approach and academic requirements to suit the needs of the student.

Lisa was identified with ADHD in elementary school. She was strong-willed, emotionally reactive and hypertalkative. When ADHD was mentioned, teachers and principals responded that she performed above grade-level, but was a discipline problem at times. Her parents were admonished to provide more structure and discipline at home. A private evaluation revealed an IQ at the 99th percentile, an ability level that certainly wasn't reflected in Lisa's school performance. She attended private schools for three years, along with private tutoring for mild learning disabilities. Lisa excelled in the gifted and talented program in which she was enrolled in 6th grade.

As social needs began to play a larger role during puberty, Lisa begged to be allowed to attend the public schools again — to be with her friends and to enjoy the much more social atmosphere of public school. Over the next several years, Lisa's performance declined. She felt lost in large classes. Her hypersocial, hypertalkative nature led teachers to react with annoyance. When her parents requested school conferences to discuss her special needs, they were admonished for Lisa's irresponsibility and lack of discipline.

Despite increasing academic difficulties, Lisa intensely resisted a return to private school. At ages 13, 14 and 15 her social world defined her. Finally, in her sophomore year of high school, Lisa herself began to realize that she was throwing away her future by remaining in a school that couldn't meet her needs. Despite the painful social upheaval, Lisa agreed that she needed to remove herself from public school and from the temptations of her social life. She entered a private boarding school which offered a class size of eight or 10, which provided a structured study hall each evening, and which gave her a daily tutoring session to help her with planning, organization, and assistance with writing assignments.

Now a student at a competitive university, she receives excellent academic support for ADHD and LD. As Lisa looks back, she believes that she would never have gone on to succeed in college without the support she received in boarding school. Rather than languishing in public high school as a very bright girl who earned mediocre grades, she received the support that allowed her to work up to her potential.

Homeschooling

Homeschooling is becoming an increasingly common alternative as families are frustrated by the low morale and academic struggles that their daughter with ADHD experiences in a public school setting.

Homeschooling is not for every family, however, and needs to be carefully considered. For homeschooling to be successful, the girl with ADHD needs to live in a home that provides the necessary structure and support for her to succeed, or needs to be highly self-motivated. Even when homeschooling is successful on an academic level, parents need to be careful to balance their daughter's activities so that she does not become socially isolated and has the opportunity to participate in the extra-curricular activities available to students in the public schools.

Many parents have found a balance between the advantages of homeschooling and the opportunities available in public schools by arranging with the local public school for their child to participate in physical education, music, art, and after school clubs and sports. There are a number of structured programs that have been developed to help parents follow a homeschooling program for their child that will prepare her across the broad range of academic subjects that are typically covered by the public schools.

This homeschooling story comes from a family of three children with ADHD. Their second child, a daughter, was on the quiet, less assertive side. She did well in elementary school, where she had the benefit of small classes, but began to fall apart as she entered her junior and senior years of high school.

As their second daughter and youngest child followed along, her ADHD was easier to identify. Kay was more assertive and outgoing, like her older brother. Her parents felt that they had overlooked so much with her sister, and were careful not to make the same mistake twice. Several weeks after Kay entered the new, large public high school, she was coming home angry on a daily basis — complaining of senseless rules, of boring classes and indifferent teachers. As her misery increased week by week, her parents took note. After an especially explosive confrontation between the students and faculty about behavior in the halls between classes, Kay came home announcing that she wanted to try homeschooling. Although her parents voiced some doubts, they did not want her to repeat the pattern of frustration and failure of her older sister.

The family launched into unfamiliar territory with their youngest child. Kay, who had always been encouraged to think and act independently, researched an intern-based homeschool program, and with her parents' permission enrolled. Four years later, Kay writes:

> *My friends laughed at me when I told them I decided I was going to homeschool. I was tired of weekly meetings with my teachers (to discuss problems), of sitting in class seven hours a day, of not being with my friends. In homeschooling I could go at my own pace. My teachers were patient with me and gave me the time to finish my work. They gave me the responsibility to finish it, and had complete trust that I would get it done. Another thing is that many of my activities were hands-on. For one social studies project my mother and I visited a nonprofit agency where I learned how dogs are trained to lead blind people.*

As I explored more in depth with homeschooling, I began to realize that learning was, for me, bringing out those qualities and talents within myself. I discovered how certain herbs help different parts of the human body. I wrote poetry and short stories. I looked for whatever made my blood sizzle and I did that.

Right now I'm at a two-year college studying various courses to get my two-year degree. Homeschooling led me to where I am right now and it was the best decision I've ever made.

Kay, like many bright, strong-willed girls with ADHD, was able, through homeschooling, to spend her energy making choices and working toward a future that suits her interests and her strengths. In a public school setting, where she felt bored and frustrated, she may have misspent that same energy battling the system and learning little.

Very little research has been done on the effectiveness of homeschooling for students with ADHD; however, one preliminary study of a small group of students with ADHD [24] demonstrated that they advanced further in both reading and math than the typical student in the public school environment from which these homeschooled students had come. The gains were attributed to the opportunity for 1:1 teaching in the home environment.

Homeschooling isn't for every family, or for every student with ADHD, but it offers the possibility of providing both the structure and the flexibility that are so often the key to success for a student with ADHD.

BRINGING IN OTHER PROFESSIONALS TO SUPPORT GIRLS WITH ADHD

Ideally, all of the necessary academic supports would be provided for girls with ADHD by the public school system. But, realistically, this is unlikely to happen. Parents of girls with ADHD need to work hard to bring the public school system into the loop in recognizing and helping their daughter with ADHD, but should not expect that all needs can or will be met at school.

Educational diagnostician

As has been mentioned earlier, when parents suspect that their daughter may have ADHD, but the teacher(s) do not recognize a problem, perhaps their best option is to elect to have their daughter evaluated by a private expert in the area of ADHD. This individual may be a clinical psychologist, a neuro-psychologist or an educational diagnostician. While the testing should contain standard, well-recognized tests in order to document an ADHD diagnosis, the most critical and useful part of the test report is the list of recommendations regarding treatment, educational needs and accommodations. The parent can then return to the school with a documented disability and commence the process by which an individual educational plan (IEP) or 504 plan (so called because of Section 504 of the Rehabilitation Act) can be developed to meet their daughter's educational needs in the school system. Often it can be helpful if the professional who conducted the evaluation accompanies the parent to the school meeting, to explain and discuss the recommendations in the report.

Tutor

ADHD traits, combined with years of self-doubts and low self-esteem, can lead girls with ADHD to shy away from challenging courses, or to assume, if such courses are required, that they will do poorly in them. Even when there is no evidence of a learning disorder in a particular subject, a girl with ADHD may greatly benefit from working one-on-one with a tutor. A tutor can support girls with ADHD in particular areas of weakness such as math, written language, or memory. She can also help her to develop the organizational and general study skills she'll need as academic demands increase in middle and high school.

Coach

Even when a girl with ADHD is bright enough to compensate academically, her ADHD may impact her in profound ways that make school highly stressful.

> *My daughter, 13, is mind-bogglingly brilliant; she knocks the top off of every standardized test, with seventh grade College Board scores of over 1200, but is unable to keep track of assignments, notebooks, lab work. She is so disorganized that we have to make a special trip to empty out her locker once a week, so she'll have a coat or sweatshirt for the following Monday.*

A girl like this could greatly benefit from specialized coaching that can help her to become better organized and less forgetful. Coaching, unlike tutoring, focuses on setting concrete goals such as habit development, and supporting the girl to follow-through on a daily basis until habits of planning and organization have become established.

Coaching for children and teens with ADHD is a profession that emerged in the mid-1990s and that has proven to be an excellent tool to help students compensate for typical ADHD patterns of disorganization and forgetfulness.

CONCLUSION

The responsibility falls upon the parents of a daughter with ADHD to try to ensure that she receives the educational support that she needs and that her full potential is reached. Parents must first become strong advocates for their daughter and then teach their daughter to become a strong advocate for herself. As we've seen in the several clinical vignettes introduced in this chapter, sometimes even strong advocacy within the public school system will not suffice. Some families will choose to opt for alternatives, either private schooling or homeschooling, to avoid potentially damaging situations.

The most critical issue for girls with ADHD is that they are identified so that they may receive appropriate support, accommodations, and treatment. The potential of so many girls is wasted because they are dismissed or overlooked. Teachers, very understandably, will have a more difficult time identifying the less-obvious behaviors of many girls with ADHD. Girls with ADHD who are functioning on grade level, but whose potential is far above their peers, are likely to be overlooked in a public school system which already feels stretched beyond capacity in its attempt to meet the diverse needs of many students. More professional teacher and parent education is necessary before the identification and adequate accommodation and support of girls with ADHD becomes routine in our public classrooms.

CHAPTER TEN

Effective Approaches for Managing ADHD

ADHD IS A COMPLEX CONDITION that pervades almost every aspect of a girl's life. We have used the term *management* rather than *treatment* in this chapter because ADHD is not a condition that is treated and cured. It is a condition that one is born with and that one lives with to a greater or lesser extent throughout one's life. The family in which a girl grows up, the school environment, and the life choices that she makes will all have a profound impact upon how she is affected by ADHD.

We've organized this chapter using a *parents first* approach to emphasize that ADHD is a disorder that must be addressed by parents within the context in which a girl lives. While all manner of therapies may be helpful in dealing with certain aspects of ADHD, the first step is for parents to take a leading role in helping their daughter. With guidance from professionals, parents need to develop a deep understanding of how their daughter is affected by ADHD, and then help her to develop a realistic, positive, constructive view of herself. Parents need to create a home environment in which their daughter can build the skills, self-understanding, and self-confidence to become successful at home, at school, and in social relationships. Medication and/or ADHD-focused psychotherapy or other supports can be helpful, but the family's understanding and support is critical to creating a positive outcome.

Marcel Kinsbourne, M.D. summarized it best when he wrote that ADHD management should target *quality of life*, not just reduction of ADHD symptoms.[1] Too often, there is an overemphasis on in-school behavior and academic performance, while a girl's overall quality of life is ignored. One of the most critical quality of life issues faced by many girls with ADHD is the repeated negative interpersonal exchanges she experiences with peers, with parents, and with teachers. Over time, these negative messages are gradually internalized to form her self-image. Negative messages can permanently damage self-esteem. Not surprisingly, one of the first ADHD gender differences identified was that females had a more negative self-image than males with ADHD.[2] Parents can play a powerful role in developing and supporting their daughter's confidence and self-esteem.

BEYOND MEDICATION

Too often, parents and teachers think first of stimulant medication as the primary treatment for ADHD. In 1994, Stephen Hinshaw, a highly regarded ADHD researcher at UC Berkeley, wrote that medication could only provide temporary gains in academic productivity, but did not, in his view, improve children's long-term academic and social functioning. His doubts were drowned out by the findings of the large, multisite MTA study in 1999,[4] which concluded that stimulant medication was superior to other treatment approaches used in the study, while the behavioral treatment provided produced only modest advantages for non-ADHD symptoms.

In early 2014, an article was published in the New York Times in which the author, Alan Schwartz, reported the results of interviews of many of the original MTA study researchers that belatedly echoed Hinshaw's misgivings about the efficacy of stimulant medication. They expressed regret for earlier claims about the benefits of medication treatment alone, following later findings that medication only addresses short-term symptom reduction, but ignores issues such as academic success, functioning in the home, social functioning and general well-being.[5]

We fully recognize the effectiveness of medication as part of an overall treatment plan and devote Chapter Eleven to a discussion of medications used in treatment of ADHD. We want to help parents and other professionals to move away from a polarizing debate about medication vs. alternatives to medication. Instead, the discussion should focus on developing a treatment plan that focuses on improving cognitive functioning and quality of life that may or may not include medication.

In this chapter, we will introduce a range of approaches to help girls with ADHD manage not only ADHD symptoms, but also the related conditions that often accompany ADHD. In all treatment approaches, the goal is to help girls with ADHD feel and function well in every aspect of their lives.

CATCH IT EARLY

Early intervention is the key to successful ADHD treatment. Early intervention is the insurance that non-adaptive coping patterns will not become entrenched, and that other symptoms will be less likely to develop secondary to ADHD. Above all, the earlier that identification and intervention can begin, the less damage will be done to a girl's developing sense of self. That being said, however, it is never too late to diagnose and treat ADHD.

HELPING PARENTS TO HELP THEIR DAUGHTERS WITH ADHD

If a girl with ADHD feels understood and supported within her family, she can begin to transfer the skills and strategies that she develops at home to the greater world. But first, we must help parents in order that they can then, in turn, help their daughters to grow in confidence and self-esteem.

PROCESSING THE ADHD DIAGNOSIS

For many parents, some time may be needed to understand and fully accept that their daughter is different and requires special considerations. During this time many feelings may arise — relief, overwhelm, frustration about prior misdiagnoses, depression, fear about the future, and even the stages of a grief reaction, mourning the loss of a normal child. Changing their expectations for their child, and then communicating those new expectations to others, is a stressful and rarely linear process. Parents will stumble through this journey at their own rate. For each parent, different aspects of the ADHD picture will produce blind spots. Well-meaning extended family can place additional pressure on a parent. And to make the process even harder, the parents need to present a united front to their child. All this takes work, and many parents can benefit from working with an ADHD expert who can guide them through this maze of feelings toward a position of acceptance, understanding and constructive support.

PARENT-CHILD COMMUNICATION ISSUES

Parent-child communication, which often has been strained to the breaking point before a diagnosis, can definitely be improved to minimize the frequency and intensity of family discord. Once parents begin to understand ADHD, they may erroneously feel that they always must be understanding and avoid feeling angry at their daughter. These parents need to understand that it is absolutely normal to be angry at one's child from time to time, and that it doesn't mean the parents don't love her enough. Parents shouldn't feel guilty about their anger. To work through these feelings, parents will need to separate their daughter's identity from the brain wiring that affects her. Above all, keeping a sense of humor about various family patterns and traits will go far to dispel the tension that can build up within families.

LEARNING AS A FAMILY TO REFRAME ADHD

Parents can help their daughters by learning to validate their daughter's experience and separate her identity from the ADHD label. She isn't ADHD, she *has* ADHD, and she also has many traits, strengths, and skills. Reframing her identity does not deny the problematic aspects of ADHD, but focuses on her unique strengths and aptitudes, and celebrates the creativity and spontaneity that springs from her often non-linear thinking.

PARENT SUPPORT GROUPS

In order to support their daughters, parents of girls with ADHD may also need to seek support for themselves. One of the most important results of participating in a parent support group is that parents who generally feel isolated by their difficulties have their experiences validated and normalized. These groups can provide an opportunity to obtain detailed and knowledgeable information about behavior management and other effective parenting techniques. In support groups, parents may also be able to describe a certain dilemma and brainstorm possible solutions. Groups like CHADD (Children and Adults with Attention Deficit Disorder — www.chadd.org) offer lectures, a lending library of books and videos, and lists of resources. Above all, parents who had been struggling alone in confusion and humiliation will find themselves immersed in a supportive network of parents who can readily relate to their challenging experiences.

DO TRY THESE AT HOME!

Overall parenting style has a massive impact on the success of any ADHD intervention program: those parents who can anticipate problems, choose their battles wisely, stay calm, consistent, and communicate acceptance are far more likely to enjoy collaboration with their daughter to help her manage the challenges of ADHD. Parents may need the support and guidance of an ADHD professional as they learn to implement and maintain changes in parenting style, but the ultimate responsibility for the effectiveness of these approaches lie with the family. Here are some ways to get started.

Begin with understanding

The single most essential factor in achieving successful management of ADHD is to develop a working knowledge of ADHD as a family. An in-depth understanding of the diagnosis and its impact provides a context for interpreting non-adaptive behaviors that sometimes seem to defy logic. The girl — as well as her parents, siblings, extended family, and teachers — need to appreciate the fallout resulting from her chronic struggle to self-regulate. As parents gain insight into their daughter's behaviors, their accusations and anger will gradually yield to declarations of support and compassion. As negative feedback decreases, so will sadness and shame, and the girl's damaged sense of self can begin to heal. Understanding the factors driving undesirable behavior, however, does not excuse it. Everyone in the family must understand that ADHD is an explanation, not an excuse. The girl with ADHD and her parents all need to work together to find better ways to reduce and manage challenging behaviors.

Create an ADHD-friendly family

One of the most powerful interventions a family can undertake is to create an environment at home in which ADHD is understood and supported. Living well with ADHD is a family affair. If one parent also has ADHD, he or she can become a role model by working to make positive changes in his own life. The parent and daughter can collaborate on finding ways to reduce ADHD challenges at home and work together to build a supportive family environment.

An ADHD-friendly family [6] is one that:

- Accepts and supports all family members, foibles and all.
- Works to understand individual differences.
- Looks for ways to simplify routines and reduce over-commitments.
- Problem solves together instead of assigning blame.
- Doesn't sweat the details, but stays focused on what's most important.
- Responds with patience and encouragement.
- Laughs together over ADHD dilemmas.
- Spends quality time together.

INTRODUCE BRAIN-FRIENDLY DAILY HABITS AT HOME

Because ADHD is a neurobiological condition, treating ADHD should embrace any and all approaches that improve overall brain functioning. Let's begin with what we know about the conditions that either optimize or compromise brain functioning.

Sleep

Various patterns of sleep disturbance have been reported in those with ADHD and are well known to all clinicians experienced in the treatment of ADHD. Researchers have only recently turned their attention to sleep problems in those with ADHD.[7] Difficulty falling asleep as well as difficulty staying asleep is found in many with ADHD. Some researchers propose that sleep loss due to inadequate sleep or disrupted sleep may be a significant factor causing the core symptoms of ADHD, particularly inattention and hyperactivity.[8]

Given the growing evidence that sleep disturbance causes or increases ADHD symptoms, one of the most critical interventions that parents can make to help their daughter with ADHD is to foster the development of healthy sleep patterns. Given the busy, over-committed lifestyles of many families today, this is easier said than done. Girls with afternoon and evening commitments to extracurricular activities often can't begin homework until mid-evening or later, leading to late bedtimes, inadequate sleep, and difficulty arising the next morning to face their busy schedule all over again. A healthier sleep regimen would likely include: strict limits on screen time (TV, iPad, smart phone, or computer) for one hour before bed; a warm bath or shower (cooling off after a shower or bath is sleep inducing), and getting to bed at the same time each night.

(For more information on developing good sleep habits, parents can refer to the article by Kathleen Nadeau, "Getting a good night's sleep." (http://chesapeakeadd.com/adhd-articles/getting-a-good-nights-sleep-with-adhd/)

Exercise

The overall importance of regular exercise is widely accepted, however, more recent findings clarify the specific cognitive benefits of daily aerobic exercise. John Ratey, in his best-selling book, *Spark*,[9] outlined research that demonstrates that aerobic exercise increases BDNF (brain-derived neurotrophic factor), the neurochemical that supports learning and that promotes the growth of neural connections (that form when learning takes place) and also promotes neurogenesis (the creation of new brain cells). One study found that teens that exercised as little as twice weekly had a much-reduced likelihood of having ADHD symptoms.[10] Exercise also helps with sleep. By encouraging your daughter to make daily exercise a part of her life, you are promoting two of the most powerful brain-friendly daily habits at once — exercise and sleep.

Nutrition

Glucose provides fuel for the brain. When glucose levels fall, thinking becomes foggy, decision-making becomes more difficult, and ADHD symptoms increase. Research has demonstrated that children's cognition and behavior are influenced by changes in glucose levels.[11] Eating food for breakfast that is metabolized more slowly, such as eggs or oatmeal, has been shown to benefit cognitive functioning during the morning hours at school.[12, 13] To give your daughter stable glucose levels throughout the day, plan meals that avoid refined sugar and starch and make sure that she has protein with meals and snacks. For more information on good nutrition for ADHD, parents can refer to the *Kid-Friendly ADHD and Autism Cookbook*.[14] In addition, a recent study found a correlation between eating a typical Western diet and ADHD, though much more needs to be explored to better understand this finding.[15]

Stress management

ADHD symptoms tend to increase as stress levels increase. Stress can result from sleep deprivation, fatigue, hunger, frustration, anxiety, and any number of other environmental factors. One important source of stress for a girl with ADHD is the demand for executive functioning that is beyond her current capacity. Parents can help to reduce their daughter's stress levels by making sure she gets enough sleep; has adequate time to get ready for school each morning; eats a protein rich breakfast that will prevent mid-morning hunger; and has healthy snacks after school when glucose levels can drop quickly. Furthermore, exercise is a well-established stress reducer.[16]

One stress reducer that is often overlooked is the simplification of the daily schedule by reducing unnecessary complications and commitments. Children today live in a busier, over-committed, more competitive environment than they did a generation or more ago. Parents and children are stressed as they rush through their days with both parents typically working full-time while trying to juggle pick-ups and drop-offs of children from various activities. Girls with ADHD who feel overwhelmed may need help in cutting back on commitments. Trying to keep up with sports, lessons, clubs, playdates, and countless extracurricular activities with their friends, often sends a girl with ADHD into overload and overwhelm. So, the message to parents and girls alike is to under-do it — leaving time for R&R.

Exposure to the natural world

Interesting research on the impact of the natural world strongly suggests that hperactivity decreases and the ability to focus and sustain attention increases in relation to how much time a child spends outside in nature. The more natural the setting the better. Being able to see trees and lawns through windows can help. Going outside to a playground or sports field is even better, and spending time in the truly natural world — in the woods on a hike, seems to help the most. These findings held true regardless of age, income level, or gender.[17]

ADVOCATE FOR YOUR DAUGHTER

As the parents learn about the unique ways in which ADHD manifests itself in their daughter, they are in the best position to communicate this knowledge to her teachers. Parents need to understand that this task falls upon their shoulders. As their daughter's advocate, they are the only ones who can alert the teachers, guidance counselors, and administrators to her special needs.

Many parents speak with the teachers of the core subjects; however, it is also prudent to speak with the teachers of special subjects (art, music, gym, computers, and so on). Some feel that this is unnecessary because those teachers do not teach academic subjects. But because these are the more novel and less structured activities, their less predictable format can be especially challenging for a girl with ADHD. In addition to initially informing the teachers, open communication and regular consultations will keep parents abreast of developing patterns of behavior, so that problems can be identified and discussed within the ADHD framework, before they escalate.

HELP FROM PROFESSIONALS

Family therapy

By viewing ADHD as something that affects everyone in the household, the family can create a more peaceful, ADHD-friendly environment within the home. Through practical problem-solving, the parents are helped to regain their authority and feel in control of the family, perhaps for the first time. Family therapy can help all family members improve communication skills so that everyone feels heard and understood; then, problem-solving can begin.

Family therapy can also help couples talk through their differences, so that they can begin to work as a mutually supportive team. Often one parent feels that they should be more strict and punitive in the face of their daughter's misbehavior or disrespect, while the other parent may over-compensate, making excuses for their daughter with ADHD. Such a parent may enable her to under-function by taking on all of the burden of reminding and assisting, even *doing* homework for their daughter when she has fallen far behind.

Family therapy is also a great place for siblings to voice feelings. Perhaps a sibling feels that all of the attention goes to the sister struggling with ADHD. Or perhaps the sibling feels that the sister gets away with everything because of her ADHD. Older siblings may feel that the younger sister with ADHD is simply an annoying bother that they try to avoid most of the time. When there are miscommunications, disagreements, and polarized positions taken in a family affected by ADHD, family therapy can be a very effective option to help the family get unstuck and work toward becoming a more mutually supportive group.

Informed acceptance and practical problem-solving

Psychoeducation, the process of helping an individual better understand and develop a more positive constructive attitude toward a particular neuropsychological challenge, is also highly beneficial in treating ADHD. Psychoeducation emphasizes helping the individual to not blame themselves, nor feel ashamed of challenges that they may experience, but rather to understand that individuals face similar challenges, not due to personal fault, but rather due to having a brain that is wired in a particular fashion.

Cognitive-behavioral approaches

The treatment of ADHD lends itself to cognitive behavioral approaches. For example, identifying patterns of thought that are self-defeating (I'm lazy; I'm stupid; I have to do things perfectly or not at all; It's hopeless.) and learning to replace them with more positive, constructive thoughts (I'll do the best I can; I'll ask for help when I need it; No one is good at everything.).

Many girls find it useful and comforting to be able to share their feelings and concerns as they process their understanding of ADHD. Individual treatment can be extremely useful as a means of helping the girl reframe her symptoms in a more positive light. The critical issue is to choose a therapist who truly understands the nuances of ADHD in girls, and works from strengths-based assessment; often a woman therapist is the best choice for a girl. Of these therapists, most will work simultaneously on practical problem-solving around issues with family, peers, school, organizations, etc., and on the underlying emotional issues.

Group treatment

For girls with ADHD, group treatment can be a very powerful therapeutic intervention. Many ADHD symptoms emerge when there are demands to process a lot of stimulation at the same time. In the controlled, low-stimulation environment of individual treatment, situations that trigger distractibility or over excitability rarely arise, making it difficult to practice new coping skills for these problems. It is the stressful classroom, the unstructured art class, or the bus ride home that are times of potential disaster. A group treatment situation serves as a safe microcosm of the social situations that a girl with ADHD may face. A great advantage is that a girl with ADHD, who may be unaware of her impact on others, can actually witness how ADHD behaviors affect others, by observing interactions among the group members. She can think through these issues much more clearly if she is not directly involved in the interaction.

For some girls with ADHD, group therapy may represent one of the first social groups to which they have belonged and in which they have been truly accepted. Being a group member can help to normalize the experience of having ADHD by demonstrating that her peers struggle with the same issues. The group also provides a safe forum for practicing skills related to social interaction, anger management, initiating conversation, and so on, with strategies geared toward behavioral change, such as planned situations, contingency management, modeling, cognitive behavioral techniques to improve self-monitoring, and positive self-talk.[19]

We are only just beginning to explore whether girls have different treatment needs than boys. One summer program for adolescents with ADHD, explored how best to build social skills. In single sex and mixed sex groups, members played various games while observers carefully noted prosocial interactions, assertiveness, self-management, compliance, physical aggression, and relational aggression. Of note, girls seemed to show more assertiveness, self-management, and compliance in all-girl settings compared to mixed sex settings. Interestingly, boys showed more socially appropriate behavior in mixed sex settings compared to all-boy settings. We hope that this is only one of many studies that will explore how best to help girls with ADHD improve functioning in all aspects of their lives.[20]

Behavior management

The main principle of behavioral treatment is that a girl's behavior can be altered by consistent consequences administered directly following her behavior. A number of different behavioral parent training programs have been developed that demonstrate encouraging results.[21] Positive consequences, like praise and attention, will reinforce a behavior that parents want to encourage. Negative consequences, like time-outs or loss of a privilege, will reduce the likelihood of unwanted behavior. The parents, with the therapist's advice, will agree on and establish a set of clear and effective rules for home life. They will create an explicit list of behavioral expectations and consequences for failing to conform, all of which will be explained to the daughter. The girl's teachers also must be aware of the plan so that they can participate with consistent messages, when necessary. Behavior/reward charts also can help a girl monitor her own changes in behavior. The long-term goal of all of these techniques is to help a girl develop as much independent control as possible, to prepare her for the natural separation process that leads into adulthood.

These techniques are logical, straightforward, and seem simple when they are first described — but that is the easy part. Putting these techniques into practice takes time, planning, self-examination, patience, and a lot of hard work on the parents' parts. For example, being completely consistent in administering this system, without anger, in all contexts, despite a pleading, crying child, is extremely difficult. Clearly, if one or both parents also have ADHD, organizing and maintaining such a system will be an extraordinary challenge. It also is important to remember that children with ADHD don't learn from behavioral reinforcement and consequences as easily as other children do.

For example, when a girl successfully puts away all of her crayons and markers after using them, the parent or teacher can say, "What a responsible job you did putting away the art supplies!" This situation-specific praise (as opposed to "What a good girl!"), accompanied by a smile and a discreet touch on the shoulder, is actually a very powerful reinforcement strategy. On the other hand, if a girl does not turn off the TV at the agreed-upon time and instead throws a temper tantrum, a parent can discipline her by putting her in a time-out. This involves establishing a quiet, safe, non-stimulating place in the house where she can be sent to cool down for an agreed-upon length of time while being deprived of family interaction and stimulation. The point of a time-out, however, is not punishment, but rather a way to provide a time to regain self-control in order to rejoin an activity or comply with a request. It is hoped that through consistent practice a girl will be able to take a time-out on her own in order to remain in control.

One promising approach developed to help children with ADHD and severe mood dysregulation is an approach that involves both the children and their parents in separate groups. In the child group, children are taught emotional regulation skills using a cognitive/behavioral approach, while in the parent group, parents are taught behavior management techniques for managing recurrent defiant behavior.[22]

Problem-solving communication training with parents and children has also shown very promising results.[23] It is particularly appropriate for middle and high school girls who may react much more positive to a collaborative approach rather than simply having negative consequences imposed for undesirable behavior.

Medication

ADHD symptoms are the result of network imbalances or insufficiencies in the neurotransmitter chemicals in the brain, particularly the dopamine system. Medication can address these neurochemical imbalances so that the girl can function better. Medication cannot cure ADHD, but it can improve the symptoms while the prescribed medication is active at adequate doses. Medication does not control the child, but rather allows the child to have more control over how she functions and who she can be. See Chapter Eleven for a full discussion of pharmacological treatment for ADHD girls.

Coaching

A coach can work one-on-one with a girl on a regular basis to help her reach her goals. Coaching is a partnership with someone who can help her learn to do the things she needs to do. A coach can help her become aware of how she functions, learns, manages her time, and make choices. Then, utilizing this unique profile of her strengths and weaknesses, the coach can help her expand her repertoire of automatic behaviors by providing the opportunity for consistent, supervised practice of skills. A coach, whether in person or over the phone, gets involved on the nitty-gritty level and helps a girl with the executive functioning difficulties that are so central to ADHD including: planning her time, setting priorities, organizing assignments, breaking down tasks, and developing effective study skills. In addition, a coach serves as a cheerleader and sounding board, as well as a provider of detailed feedback.

For teens, a coach also can help to develop a set of long-range goals, as well as explicit plans for meeting those goals. After identifying a girl's personal roadblocks to success, a coach can also work with her on developing self-advocacy skills. When the struggle between parent and daughter over academics or other responsibilities becomes a central and harrowing aspect of their relationship, it is time to consider ways for the parent to step back while another adult (coach/mentor/tutor) performs the skills-training and supervisory functions of a parent, without the parents' intense emotional investment. In that way, a coach can broaden the support network and enlarge the safety net so that the parent-child relationship can become less control-oriented and more rewarding.

Computerized brain training

There are many companies that have developed brain training software over the past 10 to 15 years. On the surface, it's a very appealing idea — it can be done at home or at school, and is relatively inexpensive. And there is an assumption that children will feel more attracted to a computer game. Cogmed^{tm} is a computerized brain training program that was originally developed in Sweden where it was used extensively in public schools. In recent years, Cogmed^{tm} has come to the United States. While Cogmed^{tm} cites numerous research articles demonstrating the positive impact of Cogmed^{tm} on working memory and attention,[24,25] other studies have found that the gains shown in Cogmed^{tm} don't transfer to functioning in daily life, in particular, in improvement of academic performance.[26]

Mindfulness training

Mindfulness Meditation is a very low-tech type of brain training which focuses on a single thing (the breath, a candle flame) and repeatedly brings the attention back to the original point of focus as soon as the individual notices his mind wandering. There have been numerous brain studies of Buddhist monks in meditation that show this can be an incredibly powerful tool. More recently, mindfulness meditation has been developed as a primary treatment of adult ADHD by psychiatrist Lydia Zylowska at UCLA,[27] with a significant body of research to demonstrate its impact on increasing focus and reducing ADHD symptoms.

Mindfulness training has also been used experimentally in a number of school settings with very positive reports from teachers and students alike, that a few moments of mindfulness meditation can help students to feel peaceful, calm and focused.[28] Even very young children have benefited from mindfulness training, using a stuffed animal that serves as their focal point. Placed on their abdomen as they lie down, the stuffed animal rising and falling on their abdomen allows them to engage in a few moments of mindfulness, as they slowly breathe in and out.[29]

Executive functioning training

As the importance of executive functions receives more and more notice, systems or programs to help children build EF skills have been developed. Executive functions are those skills needed to plan, execute, and complete a task or project. EF skills are defined differently in different publications, but generally include skills in time management, organization, planning, self-monitoring, working memory, and the skills involved in initiating, maintaining effort, and completing a task. A more thorough discussion of executive functioning can be found in Chapter Eight.

Some researchers in the ADHD field have commented that children with ADHD don't lack the knowledge about what to do; they simply lack the motivation or drive to do many tasks. A very interesting project conducted with 3rd through 5th grade students was designed to test this theory.[30] Children that were found to have executive functioning deficits were referred to a program to improve their EF skills. Children were randomly assigned to one of three groups: a waiting list, an 8-week skills-based program focusing on organization, planning, and time management; or a program where no skills were taught, however, desirable goal attainment was rewarded by parents and teachers. The findings of this project showed much stronger gains in organization, time management, and planning skills in the group that actively taught these skills and guided the children in practicing them. These gains were reported by both parents and teachers. Measurable gains were still present many months later.

This is very encouraging news, as a brief, eight-week group training experience is highly affordable and could even be offered as an after-school activity. It also suggests that this kind of skills-based teaching of OTMP (organization, time management, and planning) skills could be adapted to a general classroom setting.

TREATING ASSOCIATED DISORDERS

ADHD treatment can only be truly effective if all coexisting disorders are addressed as part of a comprehensive treatment plan. Generally, the later a girl is diagnosed, the more likely it is that she will suffer from some type of emotional or psychiatric difficulty, in addition to her ADHD. Psychiatric or developmental conditions coexisting with ADHD are quite common, existing in almost 50% of children with ADHD.[31] These coexisting disorders can alter the symptoms, pattern, course, treatment, and prognosis for a girl's ADHD. Since other disorders can confound the presentation of symptoms, one disorder may be more obvious than another, and the full diagnosis may emerge over a period of time in psychotherapy.

The tendency to internalize symptoms makes ADHD girls far more prone to develop a coexisting mood disorder, which can include dysthymia (chronic low-level depression), major depressive disorder, bipolar disorder, anxiety disorders, eating disorders, substance abuse disorders, and somatization disorders. For many girls, a history of chronic social and academic failure often leads to an escalating pattern of low self-esteem, irritability, demoralization, and learned helplessness.

Mood disorders

A girl with ADHD in childhood suffers later from major or clinical depression and anxiety disorders at much higher rates (20-25%) than a boy with ADHD (3-8%).[32] The likelihood of developing such a disorder increases dramatically in the adolescent years, especially in the case of the primarily inattentive presentation, which can so easily evade detection.[33] If ADHD remains untreated until the teen years, girls seeking help for their unhappiness may present with the symptoms of anxiety or depression, which may be easier to spot than the ADHD symptoms. It is common to have girls with ADHD treated for an extended time for these coexisting diagnoses, without success. Anecdotal reports suggest that a growing number of clinicians are recognizing ADHD in women whom they are treating for depression or anxiety. Often ADHD is considered as a possibility after depression and/or anxiety have been addressed, yet patterns of overwhelm and disorganization persist. Unfortunately, it remains rare that the typical psychotherapist has the knowledge and experience to integrate effective ADHD treatment into their therapeutic approach.

Medication regimens to address depression and ADHD are common. Some physicians prescribe an atypical antidepressant that may address both issues at once; however, many physicians find that treatment is more effective if a combination of an antidepressant is prescribed along with a psychostimulant. For more information on medication to treat these coexisting conditions, please refer to Chapter Eleven.

Depression can also be secondary to ADHD, in other words, in reaction to it. Sometimes such depression has been referred to as *demoralization*, in response to the frequent frustrations and disappointments associated with untreated ADHD.[34] In these cases, girls can often be helped very effectively by introducing daily exercise, careful attention to adequate sleep, educational supports, social engineering to increase positive social interactions, and stimulant medication.

Anxiety disorders

Anxiety disorders are another common coexisting diagnosis for girls with ADHD, especially in the predominantly inattentive presentation.[35] Anxiety may express itself as separation anxiety disorder, panic disorder, overanxious disorder, avoidant disorder; social phobia, other specific phobias, or obsessive compulsive disorder. Furthermore, expressions of anxiety can change throughout the developmental process, and anxiety and mood disorders can coexist along with the ADHD diagnosis. In some cases, the stimulant medication often used to treat ADHD symptoms can exacerbate anxiety symptoms; in other cases, the stimulant may produce symptoms of agitation and jitteriness that may be confused with an anxiety disorder. Somatization disorders are quite common in ADHD girls, and are often expressed as gastrointestinal complaints and/or headaches.[36] Combined medication treatment for anxiety and ADHD is common and is often effective when combined with ADHD-focused psychotherapy and appropriate supports at home and at school.

Disruptive behavior disorders

Disruptive behavior disorders are another major source of complications for those with ADHD. Oppositional defiant disorder (ODD) is found in girls with ADHD, though to a lesser extent than in boys, and is associated with an increased risk of behavioral, academic, and interpersonal difficulties.[37] Cases of ADHD and ODD in combination are among the more difficult cases to address — at home, in school, and in treatment. The ADHD/ODD combination is characterized by very socially discordant behavior, which may render it even more distressing to parents and teachers. For example, if you ask your daughter to clean her room, a girl with ADHD might not hear you, or might forget, or might say, "I'll do it later." If you ask a girl with ADHD and ODD to clean her room, she might say, "Do it yourself if you don't like it," or "Just stay out of here, it's private, and none of your business." They often refuse to take responsibility for their actions, and instead externalize the blame onto someone else: "I didn't break that glass. Timmy did it, he always breaks everything, and he's a liar." Anger exudes from these girls, and the intensity of this feeling, like all feelings, is amplified by their ADHD.

While these types of interactions are painful and challenging, there are several steps that frustrated parents can take to reduce the level of tension in their homes. First, most therapists can help families create a highly structured behavioral system that sets firm and explicit limits for behavior, and provides specific consequences for exceeding those limits. These systems work very well as long as parents respond with the appropriate consequences calmly and consistently. Many parents, after hearing the simplicity of the plan, believe this should be a cinch. However, the *calmly and consistently* part is not as easy as it sounds. For success, parents must present an unwavering, unified front, demonstrating that they do not feel threatened and are in control. The thinking is that by having specific consequences determined in advance, parents will feel empowered that they know how to handle the situation, and they will be able to respond without anger. This response avoids the all-too-common scenario where parents resort to punishing negative behaviors out of their own outrage, "No TV for a month!" which escalates the overall tension in the parent-child relationship.

Another helpful move is to include an ADHD coach in the family's support network. Often, oppositional girls with ADHD respond most intensely to their parents, and can be far more reasonable with other authority figures, especially if there is a good fit in terms of personality styles. If the coach is responsible for working with the girl on homework and organizational issues, it diffuses the struggle between parent and child. In this way, parent and daughter are freed to have more fun interactions, where parents don't feel that they are in the role of policeman, and where the daughter doesn't feel that she needs to be on the defensive.

Conduct disorder

Conduct disorder is seen even more rarely in girls with ADHD, and involves serious antisocial behaviors such as aggression, lying, stealing, and truancy. While the oppositional defiant diagnosis always *precedes* the development of conduct disorder, in the great majority of cases, an oppositional defiant disorder does not *lead* to conduct disorder.[38] Since these families already have dealt with the problems of a girl with ADHD plus an oppositional defiant disorder, they probably have been exposed to most of the helpful techniques. It is likely that their daughter has already been identified in some way in the system, so that the parents have a network of support. The ADHD plus conduct disorder combination is probably one of the most resistant combinations to treatment, and is highly correlated with delinquency, substance abuse, and generally poorer outcomes.[39, 40] It has been shown that those girls with ADHD who do not manifest hyperactivity rarely have either of these disruptive behavior disorders, which involve impulsive acting-out behaviors. The majority of girls with ADHD, whether due to lack of hyperactivity or in response to gender-role pressure, tend much more toward the internalizing disorders, such as depression or anxiety than the externalizing disruptive behavior disorders.

Coexisting developmental disorders

Developmental disorders are another category of potential coexisting disorders seen in girls with ADHD, that include learning disabilities and speech/language disorders among many others. (See Chapter Seven for a more complete discussion of developmental disorders associated with ADHD.) Suspicion of a developmental disorder may require a consultation or assessment by a specialist in these areas, since misdiagnosis does occur. Many girls who are identified as learning disabled in school turn out to be girls with ADHD, who are underachieving so dramatically that they appear to have specific learning disabilities when they don't. On the other hand, sometimes the underachievement of a girl with ADHD is complicated by a developmental disorder in one or more of the following areas: auditory processing, visual processing, sensory integration, memory, motor coordination, or visual-motor integration. The treatment of associated developmental disorders is too large a topic to be adequately addressed in this chapter. We mention them in this chapter on treatment in order to inform parents of the frequent association of ADHD with a broad range of developmental disorders that need to be correctly diagnosed and addressed if ADHD treatment is to be successful.

Addictions

Substance use disorders frequently co-occur with ADHD. In taking a family history, it is common to find relatives with a history of substance abuse. Sometimes, substance abuse patterns develop as an adolescent seeks relief from the stress, anxiety, and low self-esteem that often result from untreated ADHD. For example, some adolescents and young adults report a pattern of smoking marijuana at the end of the day because they find it is the only thing that significantly reduces their stress level. But true addiction can occur as well to alcohol, cocaine, crack cocaine, crystal meth, and marijuana among other substances of abuse.

Treatment of ADHD and addiction can be complex. While stimulant medication may be helpful to decrease impulsivity, therefore making it somewhat more likely that a girl can maintain sobriety, the clinician must remain very vigilant because the stimulant medication itself is a potential substance of abuse in high doses. Research has found that among substance-abusing teenage girls, 50% of them also had ADHD.[41] Substance abusing girls with ADHD were found to have started abusing drugs at an earlier age and to show a greater severity of substance abuse. These girls reported a more negative self-image when not using drugs and more improvement in self-image while using drugs. This finding is critical in terms of how best to reach and help these girls. By helping them to find areas of success and working with them to improve self-esteem through self-understanding, substance abuse issues can be more effectively addressed.

Eating disorders

Eating disorders have been reported anecdotally by clinicians since the early 1990s, however, it is only recently that research has found that ADHD is a strong risk factor in developing an eating disorder.[42] Children with ADHD have twice the risk of obesity as do children without ADHD.[43] Unfortunately, the eating disorders community, in general, has not yet integrated this finding into their treatment approach. It is our clinical experience, that treatment of girls and young women with ADHD and eating disorders needs to directly address ways to reduce impulsivity, and to simplify eating plans to accommodate the difficulties with organization and planning typically experienced by girls with ADHD.

Sleep disorders

Disordered sleep patterns have long been associated with ADHD, both in childhood and adulthood; however, only recently have sleep disorders been more seriously considered as both a symptom of ADHD as well as a possible cause of ADHD symptoms.[44] There are a variety of sleep disorders that may be experienced by those with ADHD. However, one of the most common, and most problematic is that of *delayed sleep phase syndrome* (delayed sleep onset), which can greatly exacerbate ADHD symptoms due to chronic sleep deprivation. Girls with ADHD often go to sleep at an hour that does not allow them adequate sleep before rising for the following school day.

A new and very promising treatment approach for insomnia has been developed recently called Cognitive Behavioral Therapy for Insomnia (CBT-I) that helps individuals to recognize and change their beliefs about their ability to sleep.[45] This approach involves a number of techniques that are used depending upon the particular circumstances of the individual experiencing chronic insomnia, including:

- Stimulus control therapy — setting a specific bedtime and wake time, avoiding naps, using the bedroom only for sleep.

- Sleep restriction — limiting the time you spend in bed, creating sleep deprivation in the beginning, making you better able to fall asleep at a predetermined bedtime.

- Sleep hygiene — habit changes such as reducing caffeine, getting regular exercise, and building in low-stimulation wind-down time prior to bedtime.

- Sleep environment improvement — keeping the bedroom quiet and dark, no TV in the bedroom, and hiding the alarm clock from view.

- Relaxation training — a variety of techniques to calm the mind and body, including meditation, guided imagery, and muscle relaxation techniques.

- Remaining passively awake — a paradoxical approach that involves letting go of any effort to fall asleep.

- Biofeedback — wearing a biofeedback device that provides feedback about biological signs such as heart rate and muscle tension so that you can learn how to adjust them.

The most effective treatment approach may combine several of these methods and involves working with a sleep specialist, who helps you to identify the daily patterns and attitudes that interfere with sleep, so that good sleep patterns can be achieved and maintained.

DEVELOPING A COMPREHENSIVE TREATMENT PLAN

If you are the parent of a daughter with ADHD and are working with a professional who is knowledgeable and experienced in treating the special needs of girls with ADHD, you are indeed fortunate. If you have not been so lucky, you face a daunting challenge. Becoming an active advocate for your daughter means educating yourself to the point where you can educate the community about girls with ADHD in general, and about the very specific needs of your daughter. If you don't live in a metropolitan area or near a major university, you may be a lonely pioneer. While this may not be an easy role, we hope that this book helps you to understand your daughter's needs, know your rights, and obtain the supports, accommodations, and professional services that your daughter needs and deserves.

Most professionals agree that the only truly successful approach to ADHD treatment is a comprehensive multimodal team approach. The collaborative team includes the child, parents, educators, mental health professionals, and medical professionals. A collaborative team is crucial because dueling professionals can serve only to further stress, confuse, and alienate the already struggling family. A comprehensive plan should cover four areas: support and interventions for the whole family, school success, success in community activities, and effective medical treatment.

While diagnosis usually follows the form of the medical model, which focuses on illness and pathology, the treatment plan for an ADHD girl may be more effective if it stems from a strengths-based assessment. This more holistic perspective acknowledges the problem areas, but creates a treatment plan by building on the strengths of the girl and her family support system. By using the vital and healthy aspects of the family system, the family is empowered to heal itself. While professionals are essential collaborators in the process, the family is able to see that it is within their power to create an ADHD-friendly environment, custom-tailored to their daughter's needs.

The parents' roles

In any treatment plan, the role of the parents is paramount. Parents provide information and feedback to the team, observe the girl with ADHD in the widest variety of settings, dispense medications, and implement behavior-management strategies. They advocate for their daughters when their daughters are unable to do so for themselves. And, above all, no part of a treatment plan can be administered without the parents' agreement and participation; without their blessing, any treatment plan is doomed.

The teachers' roles

The teacher is responsible for facilitating the school intervention plan that has been developed. They are responsible for implementing both the regular education accommodations and the specialized modifications to maximize learning, academic achievement, and successful behavior management. Teachers also are a valuable source of feedback. They observe your daughter for a significant portion of the day, five days a week. They see how your daughter functions when you, as parents, are not present. They see the impact of medication, and can give precise information about when the medication seems to kick in, and when it may be wearing off. By being educated and sensitized to your daughter's differences, they will have a basis for interpreting her behaviors and intervening earlier in a difficult situation.

The psychologist's role

The child psychologist can diagnose and assess the disorder using a combination of checklists, interviews, testing instruments, reports from other professionals, and clinical observations. If an assessment of general cognitive functioning is necessary, a psychologist can administer the indicated tests and interpret the data in terms of strengths and weaknesses, as well as clarify the cognitive style of the girl with ADHD. They also consult with teachers concerning educational and behavioral interventions, conduct individual and group therapy as well as skills training, and consult with parents around effective home management issues and emotional issues that may arise. They also assist in day-to-day medication monitoring, and issue-by-issue problem solving. They provide support and encouragement for the daughter and her parents.

The physician's role

The pediatrician/general practitioner rules out other medical explanations for the symptoms observed in girls, and gets a baseline description of her physical status and developmental history before any medication treatment is begun. When medication is indicated, a pediatrician, general practitioner, or child psychiatrist can prescribe it. When there are coexisting diagnoses that also may require pharmacological intervention, a psychiatrist or other sub-specialist may be the more appropriate professional to join the team.

EXAMPLES OF COMPREHENSIVE TREATMENT PLANS

Many parents have shared descriptions of their daughters with us. We are using four of these descriptions to illustrate some of the many ways that ADHD can play out at each developmental stage. These four girls had just been diagnosed, and their overwrought parents asked us, "What's next?"

AMANDA, AGE FOUR DESCRIBED BY HER FATHER

Amanda was active even when she was in her mother's belly. As a toddler, she never stopped moving, never napped, but would just fall asleep right in the middle of an activity. By the time she was three, she had stitches in her forehead from various adventures. Now, at age four, two different nursery schools said that they are not an appropriate placement for Amanda. She still uses her pacifier to go to sleep at night and has great difficulty falling asleep at a reasonable hour. It's impossible to get her dressed in the morning. We try to get her to dress herself, but we end up doing it ourselves. Sometimes she hugs other kids so hard that she knocks them down. Amanda has demonstrated coordination problems, gross motor (she couldn't hop or skip), and fine motor (she pressed so hard on the crayon that it broke in two). The kindergarten we were considering recommended that Amanda start a pre-K program in the fall, and put off kindergarten another year.

Amanda's treatment plan might include:

- An examination by a developmental pediatrician or pediatric neurologist to confirm the ADHD diagnosis, and to rule out other possible causes for her behavior.

- A consultation with a child psychologist who can evaluate Amanda's cognitive, behavioral, and emotional functioning. With that information, the psychologist can provide parent counseling as necessary and can assist the parents in finding a preschool setting that can accommodate Amanda's needs, interfacing with the teacher as necessary.

- An evaluation by the Committee on Preschool Special Education (CPSE) to determine if Amanda meets the criteria for receiving support services, such as placement in a therapeutic nursery setting, which can offer a very low child-teacher ratio, and is well suited for addressing individual needs.

- Amanda's parents should make every effort to create a structured and predictable home environment, including firm adherence to a behavior modification plan.

- Develop a daily routine that includes a lot of physical exercise so that Amanda can expend excess energy in a safe and socially acceptable way. Consider enrollment in a Gymboree-type program that targets different muscle groups.

- Amanda's parents should consider joining the local CHADD chapter (Children and Adults with Attention Deficit Disorders) that has monthly meetings offering parent support, speakers, a lending library of ADHD materials, and a list of area resources.

ALLISON, AGE EIGHT
DESCRIBED BY HER MOTHER

It was never easy to hug Allison. When she was upset, she curled up into a ball and sat in the corner. No talking, no crying, just rocking herself. She'd ignore you like you weren't there. She seems unhappy a lot of the time, but she doesn't complain about anything special. I wonder if a girl of eight can be depressed. Allison likes to stay back on the fringes of things, although I guess she'd join a game if someone came up and asked her. Her teacher says she does OK on her work, but often misses the details of the teacher's instructions. She won't speak up in class, and avoids eye contact.

She still drags around this baby blanket that's in shreds, and sucks on the corner of it. She loves soft things like that; she's only got one pair of pajamas she's willing to wear. She has one friend across the street who's two years younger, and all they do is play computer games. Allison is such a couch potato. One thing, though: she loves to draw, and spends hours in her room with this new set of markers she got for her birthday. When I came in her room and said I really liked her drawings, she looked surprised and said, "Sometimes, it feels like I'm no good at anything." That really bothered me, because I used to feel the same way when I was a kid.

Allison's treatment plan might include:

- Teacher implementation of interventions designed by psychologist to address inattentive symptoms and shyness.
- Consult with a psychologist about psychotherapy, which might include cognitive reframing techniques to improve self-esteem. Because of her genetic loading and her tendency to internalize, Allison should be considered at risk for depression and should be assessed periodically.
- Standardized test battery if problems in cognitive functioning are suspected.
- Find a structured extracurricular activity of high interest to Allison that can provide a circumscribed opportunity for peer interaction.
- Focus on one-on-one play dates with a pre-arranged ending time and parental guidance.
- Consider getting a small furry pet (gerbil, hamster) to help her work through her tactile defensiveness.
- Help her focus on her art as an *island of competence* by offering her art lessons, keeping her supplied with materials, and framing some of her work and hanging it up in the house.

KAREN, AGE 12
DESCRIBED BY HER MOTHER, WHO ALSO HAS ADHD

Karen is so popular! She has shiny dark hair and dark eyes that flash when she smiles. She's always on the phone, giggling with her friends, boys and girls. She's the one to come up with crazy ideas like, "Let's call up each boy in the class, and when they answer, we'll hang up!" But the way she talks, with so much charisma, she gets everyone going. She just loves being the center of attention, and I always say she should be an actress. She gets in trouble for talking in class; last week, she made a nasty comment about the teacher, but the teacher heard it because Karen always talks really loud and really fast. But even when she goes to detention, she has fun. She doesn't always remember homework assignments and, when she does, she finishes really quickly so she can get back to her friends. She goes into town every day after school and hangs with a bunch of kids near the pizza place. It drives me nuts that she always comes home late, no matter what I do. Karen just started 'going out' with Mike — he's in 8th grade — so she thinks they are THE cool couple and that school's just not that important. What can I do? She's already boy crazy!

A sample treatment plan for Karen might include:

- Parent training sessions to learn techniques for limit-setting.
- Frank parent-child discussions about safe sex and the risk of pregnancy. Also, parents should be explicit about their values and expectations about smoking, drugs, and alcohol.
- ADHD group for Karen to learn/practice self-monitoring skills.

- Regular consultation with teachers, encouraging frequent contact between parent and teacher.

- Discussion of puberty and its impact on ADHD symptoms, facilitated by a professional.

- Use of a coach to keep schoolwork on track, and remove mother from that struggle.

- Consult with a psychiatrist for an evaluation for medication.

- Buy a beeper/cell phone for Karen.

- Link privileges, such as phone and social time, to school performance.

- Consider transfer to private school with more supervision.

- Structure after school and weekend time so that socialization is under adult supervision.

LINDSAY, AGE 16
DESCRIBED BY HER MOTHER

Lindsay is a terrific girl, just terrific. She studies hard, and stays up late doing it. And she usually gets good grades. That's how I got through law school. But she worries a lot about school, and works really slowly. Another problem is that she's a lazy reader; she starts to read and then falls asleep on her book. Lately, she's been losing weight, which was fine at first. It's better to control food than to let it control you, right? But now she seems obsessed with not eating. And all the clothes she buys now are either black or white. She says she doesn't have any big decisions getting dressed in the morning because everything matches now. She must have at least six pairs of black pants, each one in a smaller size than the one before. I don't like to argue with her because when she finally loses it, watch out! She doesn't have a lot of friends, but she has one best friend, Jody. Believe it or not, they love to play Scrabble, but Jody hates it when Lindsay takes forever to put a word down and then straightens all the tiles. I would never have thought ADHD could look like this.

A sample treatment plan for Lindsay might include:

- Evaluation for anorexia and other comorbid conditions, such as obsessive-compulsive disorder by a psychiatrist, who can explain the impact of hormonal fluctuations on ADHD, rule out other explanations for weight loss, and evaluate Lindsay for medication.

- Consult with a psychologist about individual treatment.

- Find a therapeutic peer support group so that Lindsay can practice socialization skills.

- Teach Lindsay self-advocacy skills.

- Understand that reading difficulties are common for girls with ADHD, and not due to laziness; get books on tape.

CONCLUSION

Fortunately, there are parents who have gone before you, working fiercely at times, to create a supportive and consistent ADHD-friendly environment in which their daughters can thrive. Each of these families served as strong advocates for their daughters. Each, in their unique way, worked to help their daughters find a path that would lead her to recognize and respect her differences, so that she can develop the best of herself. As parents, professionals, and teachers following in the wake of these pioneering efforts, we can benefit from their experience. We each can do our part to extend their efforts to make life in the family, school, and community more accepting of their differences and more appreciative of the talents and abilities of these girls.

Clearly, every girl with ADHD is unique. In fact, there are few disorders that can present with such widely disparate symptoms while having the same underlying neurological picture. Age, temperament, family environment, heredity, interests, and abilities all contribute to the unique experience of each girl with ADHD. And in order to maximize each girl's success, her needs require specialized and individualized interventions. The paths carved out by the girls and their families in this book are examples of possible symptom pictures, and may not be suitable plans for every girl with ADHD. Our hope is that we have presented varied and flexible models for parents, professionals, and teachers to consider and adapt. Ultimately, it is the goal of that committed team to help these girls reach their fullest potential, with their self-esteem intact, and pride in the person they are becoming.

CHAPTER ELEVEN

Medication for ADHD
Making the Decision Isn't Easy

FOR MORE THAN 50 YEARS, stimulant medications have been used to treat ADHD. Thousands of studies have been conducted demonstrating both safety and efficacy of stimulants at reducing the symptoms of ADHD. Yet, when it comes to making a decision to place your daughter on medication for ADHD, the science becomes personal and numerous questions invariably arise. In addition to gathering information about the various medications and side effects, your expectations for what medication can do should also enter into the treatment decision.

THE FACTS

Stimulant medications have been shown in numerous studies[1,2] to effectively reduce the core behavioral symptoms of ADHD (inattention, impulsivity and/or hyperactivity) with 65% to 75% of children and adolescents being shown to be responders.[3] When these core symptoms are normalized, children with ADHD may show improvements in several areas including social skills, homework completion, and overall level of impairment. In addition, use of stimulants was found to be associated with significantly higher self-esteem. In one study, children with ADHD taking stimulants reported feeling smarter and more accepted by peers than children that were unmedicated. Children with ADHD and ODD reported feeling better behaved when medicated. There also seemed to be a dose effect with children taking higher doses of stimulants reporting higher self-esteem.[4]

However, a significant number of children fail to show meaningful improvement in these important areas even when symptoms are reduced. Medications don't teach organizational, social, or other executive functioning skills, and even with symptom normalization, overall academic performance may not improve even though issues such as homework problems may improve.[5] Unfortunately, many parents of children with ADHD think that taking medications alone will solve all of their child's problems.

In most people with ADHD, medications to treat the core symptoms should not be used alone but in combination with other supports to improve skills and address psychological and emotional problems. The availability and effectiveness of alternative therapies such as cognitive behavioral therapy, behavior management techniques, coaching, social skills training, and psychotherapy should all be considered before making a final decision regarding medication. In the end, after careful consideration of all of the aspects of the question of whether to give your daughter medication for ADHD, one fact will remain – most girls with ADHD need a comprehensive treatment plan (CTP) to effectively deal with all aspects of their ADHD and with any coexisting condition (see discussion of CTP below).

After doing your homework and getting all of your questions answered, you may decide that medication is not what you choose for your daughter at this time. That's okay, but it's important to keep an open mind and to make sure that your decision is based on facts, not fiction and fear. Over time, situations change and the possibility of adding medication as part of a total treatment program may need to be revisited. Most parents only want what is best for their daughter. It's hoped that we can help in this process by providing facts and answering your most urgent questions about using medication to treat ADHD in girls.

COMPREHENSIVE TREATMENT PLAN (CTP)

Both the American Academy of Pediatrics and the American Academy of Child and Adolescent Psychiatry, in their treatment guidelines to physicians, recommend stimulant medication alone or in combination with behavioral and other interventions as part of a comprehensive treatment plan to improve ADHD symptoms for children and teens with ADHD.[6,7] This individualized CTP should also take into account the chronic nature of ADHD and consider the most recent evidence concerning other effective therapies. The plan should establish and focus on target outcomes with frequent follow-ups to monitor progress.

CHOOSING A MEDICATION

While short-acting stimulants, those lasting 4-6 hours, have been available for over 50 years to treat ADHD symptoms, recently released longer-acting formulations of these medications that may be effective for 10 to 13 hours are preferred for the treatment of ADHD of children and teens for several reasons. First, medication that can be taken once a day, either by mouth or as a patch, is more convenient for both the child and her family. Second, a long-acting stimulant taken at home before the school day begins allows the child or teen with ADHD to preserve her privacy. Third, long-acting stimulants that maintain effectiveness throughout the day and into the evening, are beneficial for older elementary school children and adolescents who need control of ADHD symptoms for after school activities such as homework, athletics, or social activities, as well as during late day/evening driving or part-time work environments.[8, 9]

Some girls may respond better to one stimulant over another, but approximately 95% of them do improve when the correct stimulant and dose are found.[10] In each case, optimum response is usually determined by trial and error, with the caveat that if one stimulant does not work or makes other symptoms worse, another stimulant should be tried. Working closely with your daughter's health care provider to find the most effective dose with the fewest side effects is the goal of therapy. To accomplish this goal it is important to be patient, document target symptoms, monitor progress on a daily or weekly basis, and set-up a careful follow-up program with checks several times a year.

STIMULANTS

Stimulant medications used to treat ADHD belong to two classes. One class, containing methylphenidate as the primary ingredient, is known by the brand names Ritalin*tm*, Metadate*tm*, Focalin*tm*, Concerta*tm*, Daytrana*tm*, and Quillivant*tm*. Other medications belong to the class of drugs containing amphetamine. These are commonly sold as Dexedrine*tm*, Adderall*tm*, and Vyvanse*tm*. For girls who have difficulty swallowing pills, different medications offer various solutions. Some capsules (Metadate*tm*, Adderall*tm*) may be opened and sprinkled on food;[11] other medications come in a skin patch (Daytrana*tm*) or liquid (Quillivant*tm*) form. The delivery of methylphenidate into the blood stream by skin patch technology has certain advantages (ability to use a lower dose and flexibility of wear time) and has been shown to be effective in improving symptoms when compared to a placebo patch[12] or other long-acting methylphenidate preparations with 70% of participants showing improvement.[13,14]

Most frequent side effects seen in all of the stimulant medications include headache, decreased appetite, stomachache, trouble sleeping (insomnia), and irritability.[15,16] Effects of stimulants on sleep in children with ADHD included a decrease in total sleep time. It also took the children approximately an hour longer to fall asleep, although they went to bed at the same time as before taking medication.[17] Side effects do not occur in everyone taking a stimulant medication; and even if they do occur, they tend to be short-lived and to decrease over the first several months of therapy. Side effects have been found to occur in from 4% to 10% of those individuals treated with long-acting formulations. Serious side effects were reported to be very rare and no differences have been found in these side effects among the different stimulants.[18-20] Since growth disturbances have been reported during the first three years of taking medication,[21] it is now recommended that children's height and weight be monitored regularly, throughout treatment.[22]

HOW STIMULANTS WORK

In order to discuss how stimulants work, you may need to go back and review the areas of the brain and neurochemical transmitters involved in ADHD discussed in Chapter Two. Evidence from neuroimaging studies (MRI and PET) have demonstrated smaller size and impaired functioning in specific areas of the brain in those individuals with ADHD compared to non-ADHD controls.

Despite the longstanding use of stimulant medications to treat ADHD, the neural mechanisms underlying their cognition and therapeutic actions have only recently begun to be examined. Research has now confirmed that large doses of stimulants produce increases in levels of the neurotransmitters dopamine and norepinephrine.[23] In contrast, lower doses of stimulants that improve cognitive functioning are shown to not only increase neurotransmitter levels, but also improve signal processing.

One early study to give us clues as to what's going on in the brain in response to stimulants was conducted by Volkow and associates in 2002.[24] In this study they used PET scans to investigate the mechanism of action of methylphenidate in the brain. Results revealed that at therapeutic doses methylphenidate blocked more than 50% of dopamine transporters (DAT) and increased dopamine (DA) levels in the brain. They also found that the variability in methylphenidate increases in dopamine was the result of not only differences in DAT blockade but also differences in DA release in individuals. They postulated that it was these differences that resulted in the wide range of doses required to treat ADHD. In another study in adults with ADHD,[25] researchers used PET scans to look at the brain before and after several weeks of treatment and found that methylphenidate modulates brain regions associated with motor function to achieve a reduction in ADHD symptoms.

Several other studies[26-28] conducted in animals have shown that low doses of methylphenidate improves the working memory and attentional functions of the prefrontal cortex, while high doses impair working memory and produce a perseverative pattern of errors. These observations have provided the first definitive evidence that the PFC is a site of action in the cognition-enhancing and presumably therapeutic actions of low-dose psychostimulants.

NON-STIMULANTS

Non-stimulants have also been used alone or in combination with one of the stimulants to treat ADHD. These medications include clonidine (Catapres, Kapvey) and guanfacine (Tenex, Intuniv). These, too, have proven effective for the treatment of ADHD although the effectiveness is lower than for stimulants.[29] These medications can be particularly effective in children who are hyperaroused, over-vigilant, and overanxious. Intuniv can be used as an alternative to stimulants or as an adjunct to treatment when the stimulants alone don't seem to be adequately reducing the ADHD symptoms. For more information about adding Intuniv to an already existing stimulant therapy, see http://www.intuniv.com/hcp/adjunctive/efficacy.aspx. Side effects are also seen with non-stimulants and include sedation, appetite decrease, and irritability.

TREATING ADHD IN GIRLS WITH MEDICATION

Looking at medication treatment studies conducted to date, there are several statements we can now make regarding the treatment of ADHD in girls.[30,31] First, girls of all ages treated with ADHD medications had greater improvement in ADHD symptoms than girls who did not receive active treatment. Second, despite the often marked differences in ADHD presentation between boys and girls, girls treated with medications for ADHD show improvements in ADHD symptoms similar to the treatment-induced improvements seen in boys. Girls with ADHD were statistically indistinguishable from comparison boys on nearly all measures. Girls exhibited significant beneficial effects from both classes of stimulants (amphetamines and methylphenidate), with nearly all responding favorably to one or both drugs in this short-term trial. And, third, inattentive presentation is more common among ADHD girls in childhood and adolescence than in boys. Girls with this presentation showed marked symptom improvement when treated with ADHD medications.[32,33]

Studies have shown that these stimulant medications are as effective for reducing symptoms of ADHD in girls as in boys[34,35] although only a few studies have looked at the effectiveness of medications specifically in a female population. One such study looked at the treatment of adolescent girls with ADHD with long-acting methylphenidate (Ritalin LA) and compared it to placebo in controlling symptoms.[36] Results confirmed that methylphenidate was significantly more effective in reducing symptoms when compared to placebo in these girls.

In another study,[37] girls with combined type ADHD were evaluated to look at effectiveness of either long-acting Adderall XR (an amphetamine based stimulant) or atomoxetine (a non-stimulant). After an 18-day treatment period, Adderall XR was found to be significantly more effective than atomoxetine in terms of ratings of classroom behavior, attention, and academic productivity. However, both groups had a significant increase from baseline in the mean number of math problems attempted and answered correctly. Girls who received Adderall XR attempted significantly greater numbers of problems compared with those who received atomoxetine. Both medications were well tolerated. The most frequently occurring treatment-related side effects in girls receiving Adderall XR*tm* were decreased appetite, upper abdominal pain, insomnia, and headache. The most frequently occurring treatment-related adverse events in girls receiving atomoxetine were drowsiness, upper abdominal pain, vomiting, nausea, and decreased appetite.

Treating girls with ADHD is often more complicated than treating boys due to some of the gender specific issues like hormonal fluctuations and other coexisting conditions. The goal of treatment with stimulants is always to find the lowest effective dose that allows for maximal therapeutic benefits with the fewest side effects.[38] The severity of symptoms, presence of coexisting diagnosis, and the efficacy of ADHD treatment will determine the need for various drug combinations on a case-by-case basis. Parents should not be surprised if it takes a while to find the correct dose or combination of medications to effectively treat their daughter's symptoms.

STIMULANT USE IN PRESCHOOLERS

The American Academy of Pediatrics (AAP) guidelines for the treatment of preschool children with ADHD (four to five years of age) recommends parent and teacher administered behavioral therapy as first-line treatment for ADHD with the prescription of methylphenidate only if the behaviors do not improve and impairments are moderate to severe.[39] Studies of stimulant treatment and resulting side effects in preschool ADHD children ages three to six years, although not as numerous as in older children and adolescents, have now been conducted. Treatment benefits have been reported in 89% of controlled stimulant trials involving a total of 206 preschool children as reported by Connor in a review of the studies in 2002. Results indicate that in comparison with school-aged children with ADHD, there may be a greater variability of stimulant response in ADHD preschoolers. Preschool children were also reported to experience slightly more and different types of stimulant-induced side effects compared with older children although most side effects were mild in nature. This review, however, finds stimulants to meet evidence based criteria as beneficial and safe for carefully diagnosed ADHD preschool children aged three years and older.[40]

The Preschool ADHD Treatment Study (PATS), a large, multisite study, provides us with the best information to date about treating very young children diagnosed with ADHD. The results show that preschoolers may benefit from low doses of medication when it is closely monitored, but the positive effects are less evident and side-effects are somewhat greater than previous reports in older children.[41]

The preschoolers enrolled in the study ranged in age from three to five years. The children and their parents initially participated in a 10-week behavioral therapy and training course. Only those children with the most extreme ADHD symptoms who did not improve after the behavioral therapy course and whose parents agreed to have them treated with medication were included in the medication study. In the first part of the medication study, the children took a range of doses from a very low amount of 3.75 mg daily of methylphenidate, administered in three equal doses, up to 22.5 mg/day. By comparison, doses for school-aged children usually range from 15 to 50 mg total daily. The study then compared the effectiveness of methylphenidate at various doses to placebo. It found that the children taking methylphenidate had a more marked reduction of their ADHD symptoms compared to children taking a placebo, and that different children responded best to different doses. Preschoolers with ADHD may need a low dose of methylphenidate initially, but they may need to take a higher dose later on to maintain the drug's effectiveness.[42] Side effects in this younger group included emotional outbursts, difficult falling asleep, repetitive behaviors/thoughts, appetite decrease and irritability.[43]

DIAGNOSING COEXISTING CONDITIONS AND FOLLOWING TREATMENT GUIDELINES

After establishing that a girl has ADHD, the next step is to determine whether any other symptoms she manifests are secondary to the failure, demoralization, and poor self-esteem associated with ADHD or whether there is a true, coexisting condition in addition to the ADHD.[44] Once this question has been answered and the diagnoses have been clearly delineated, treatment usually follows one of two paths succinctly outlined in the American Academy of Child and Adolescent Psychiatry's guidelines for treatment.[45] If untreated ADHD, and its aftermath, is the primary cause of the symptoms seen, treatment with stimulants as part of a comprehensive program is undertaken to reduce ADHD symptoms, improve day-to-day functioning, and enhance overall well-being.

As discussed previously, anxiety, depression, mood disorders, including bipolar disorder, and obsessive/compulsive traits are common coexisting conditions seen in girls with ADHD.[46, 47] While stimulants increase attention and decrease distractibility, they may worsen some of these other conditions. How, then, is ADHD treated when another condition is present? In order to address all of the symptoms a girl with ADHD might be experiencing, varying dosage schedules and unique combinations of medications may need to be considered.

If ADHD exists with other coexisting conditions, while the use of stimulants is not contraindicated, caution may need to be exercised as stimulants may increase anxiety and OCD, and, in some girls, worsen depression. It is important then that these coexisting conditions be adequately treated in addition to the ADHD. Guidelines here recommend that in mild to moderate cases of anxiety or depression, the ADHD may be treated first, and other conditions treated later if necessary.[48] In cases where the coexisting condition is severe, the recommendation is to prioritize treatment. In the case of coexisting depression, if the depression is severe with vegetative symptoms (problems with sleeping or eating) and/or suicidal thoughts, the recommendation is to treat the depression first. In cases of bipolar disorder and ADHD, mood stabilizers will be given first and once mood is stabilized, stimulants will need to be added later to treat the ADHD.[49]

USING ANTIDEPRESSANTS FOR ADHD

Antidepressants known as selective serotonin reuptake inhibitors (SSRIs), such as Zoloft, Prozac, Paxil, etc., while effective for treating a variety of disorders including depression, obsessive-compulsive disorders, and panic, are not, in general, indicated for use as a primary drug for the treatment of ADHD symptoms. For girls with depression, OCD, panic, anxiety, and ADHD, however, the use of the SSRIs may be quite effective in combination with a stimulant. Studies looking at combined therapy for children with ADHD and coexisting conditions indicate that after inadequate response to a methylphenidate alone, treatment with both methylphenidate and fluoxetine (Prozac) reduces depressive symptoms by two-thirds, with overall improvement in functioning in about one-third in these children.[50,51]

TREATING ADHD AND BIPOLAR DISORDER

Children with ADHD, particularly adolescent girls and young women, can be diagnosed with bipolar disorder, in addition to their ADHD.[52] In these cases, it is important to be sure to differentiate the diagnosis of bipolar disorder (BPD) from ADHD and coexisting depression, which tends to be seen more commonly in females. While ADHD and bipolar disorder can co-occur, it is usually the ADHD that is diagnosed first. Once the diagnosis of bipolar disorder is made, by a professional well-trained in differentiating the symptoms of ADHD from mania and hypomania, it is imperative to treat both the bipolar disorder and the ADHD to assure improvement. In these cases, mood stabilizers are usually prescribed first for a period of several days to weeks to address the bipolar symptoms. Once the bipolar disorder is stabilized, a stimulant may be added to effectively treat the ADHD symptoms without the danger of making the bipolar symptoms worse, which can occur when treatment is undertaken with stimulants alone. Concurrent treatment for both of these conditions is imperative, and prognosis for improvement is poor if either condition remains untreated.[53]

ADHD, EATING DISORDERS, AND OBESITY

ADHD, eating disorders, and obesity have several symptoms in common. These include impulsivity, low self-esteem, and often depression. Impulsivity has been shown to be a significant factor for developing eating disorders in a study of adolescent girls with ADHD.[54] Healthy eating habits require a great deal of organization and planning skills that girls with ADHD often lack. In addition, a girl needs to self-regulate and pay attention to when she is hungry and to stop eating when she is full. Girls with ADHD may overeat for other reasons: feeling out of control and stressed from their ADHD symptoms, for stimulation when they are bored, lack of control (once they start they can't stop), or a lack of awareness of how much or why they are eating. This mindless or compulsive overeating can often result in obesity. Studies have now shown that undiagnosed ADHD may be an underlying condition in more than half the cases of significant obesity presenting at weight management clinics[55, 56] and that both female gender and not taking stimulants for ADHD symptoms increase the risk for obesity.[57]

By treating the symptoms of ADHD it is possible to address many of the issues that lead to binge eating, obesity, and other eating disorders. In an article published in the May 2005 issue of the *Journal of Women's Health*, Carolyn Dukarm, MD, an eating disorders specialist, describes six patients with bulimia and ADHD, who were treated with dextroamphetamine. All six patients reported no further episodes of binge eating and purging following treatment. In five of the six patients, ADHD had not been previously diagnosed, perhaps due to the fact that all six had the inattentive presentation of the disorder.[58] These cases, along with other recent clinical study findings and anecdotal reports, seem to confirm the association between bulimia nervosa/binge eating and ADHD in girls and women and have important clinical and therapeutic implications. Today, larger studies for the treatment for ADHD and ED with the newer long-acting stimulants are underway.

A more detailed look at the potential role of ADHD and its treatment in the management of bulimia and binge eating is described by Dukarm in her book discussing the relationship between ADHD and eating disorders. Here she states that in addition to treating the symptoms of ADHD, treatment with stimulants also decrease the urge to binge. In *Pieces of the Puzzle: The Link between ADHD and Eating Disorders*, Dukarm offers an extremely detailed diagnosis and treatment program for patients with the dual diagnosis and for the clinicians who treat them.[59]

ADHD AND PMS

PMS and its associated irritability and mood swings often need to be addressed in the adolescent girl with ADHD. If PMS is mild, lifestyle changes such as exercise, dietary modifications, relaxation and cognitive behavioral therapy may improve symptoms. In addition, for some girls with physical symptoms, non-steroidals, such as ibuprofen, may be necessary. However, more severe PMS with more symptoms may require treatment with antidepressants in the SSRI category on symptom days only. These SSRIs include Zoloft, Prozac, and Paxil.[60] Girls with ADHD, who also experience PMS or premenstrual dysphoric disorder (PMDD), may need to be treated with one of these drugs, in addition to a stimulant for their ADHD symptoms.

The picture may become even more complicated if a girl has depression, PMS, and ADHD. Rather than place her on two antidepressants, in addition to her stimulant therapy, it would seem preferable to place her on an SSRI and a stimulant. However, the prescribing physician should be aware that the SSRI dosage might need to be increased prior to menstruation to address the PMS irritability. The maintenance dose of the SSRI used to treat depression effectively may not be enough to treat the PMS symptoms, and managing these symptoms appears to be critical in some girls. Low-dose estrogen birth control pills have been used in the past to help relieve symptoms of severe PMS or PMDD, but evidence that serotonin levels in the brain are involved, has led to treatment with an SSRI for regulating mood and decreasing rage and depression that occur prior to menstruation.[61]

BRIANNA'S STORY
A COMPLEX TREATMENT CASE STUDY

Brianna's case seems typical for many girls with ADHD, who manifest anxiety-related disorders in addition to their ADHD, and illustrates the necessity to treat each symptom complex in order to effectively improve overall functioning. Brianna was at times immobilized by her OCD, panic, and anxiety which all worsened after puberty. However, with appropriate treatment, Brianna had stabilized by college, and she could manage her symptoms effectively with a little additional support.

Brianna, a beautiful, tall, dark-haired, 15-year-old, was referred during her first year in high school for evaluation of possible attention deficit disorder. At that time, Brianna reported that she had a great deal of difficulty sitting still and concentrating. She was distracted easily by both visual and auditory stimuli. Some impulsive behaviors were noted, and Brianna was known for her constant talking. Visual images and doodling would help focus Brianna during lectures, and she frequently used an outline to stay on track. She was poor at note-taking and doodled rather than taking notes in class. Brianna reported that she was a slow reader and did not like to read.

In addition to these problems, Brianna had an overly developed awareness of germs. She constantly felt that she must wash her hands, and demanded that others wash their hands before touching her or her things. She also reported that she felt unbalanced if her body was touched and she needed to have everything symmetrical. If she was touched on one side, she needed to touch her other side to feel better.

Brianna had had seizures that continued from birth until nine months of age. As a small child, she was hypersensitive to touch and textures. As a preschooler, Brianna was described as being hyperactive, messy, and having difficulty with transitions. It had always been difficult for her to fall asleep at night, and she had given up her naps early. Her family history included other family members diagnosed with tics, OCD, and auditory processing problems and her mother thought that perhaps she, too, had ADHD.

Upon completion of neurodevelopmental and educational assessments, including reports from her parents and teachers, Brianna was diagnosed as having attention deficit/hyperactivity disorder (ADHD) and obsessive compulsive disorder (OCD). Primary recommendations were for a trial of stimulant medication and counseling. Tutoring was also undertaken to improve organizational, note taking, and reading comprehension skills. It was explained to Brianna that the stimulant medication, while alleviating her difficulty with concentrating and her hyperactivity, could possibly complicate her OCD symptoms or tics.

Brianna decided that her ADHD symptoms were the most prevalent and bothersome, and the ones that she elected to treat. Alternative and additional medication interventions were also discussed at that time.

Brianna was placed on methylphenidate, and close monitoring was undertaken. Brianna and her teachers reported positive changes at school. Her germ phobia was perceived as being a little worse, or, perhaps, she was more aware of it. At home, her parents noted increased irritability and slight appetite decrease. She continued on this regime for approximately a year. At that time, Brianna reported that her OCD was getting worse and that she was more irritable and jittery. She decided that she would like to try medication to address these problems as well. She began a trial of clonidine and experienced a significant reduction in phobias, irritability, and OCD symptoms.

Over the next year, however, Brianna developed full-blown panic attacks. She began taking Prozac and used relaxation and biofeedback techniques. When her clonidine was discontinued, her OCD symptoms returned. ADHD symptoms remained under control with methylphenidate, but her grades were inconsistent because of an inability to sustain effort and remain organized at times. Brianna began to work with a coach on these issues. Panic attacks abated over the next two months. The stimulant and SSRI combination was maintained for another year. At that time, the SSRI was decreased to every other day and eventually was taken only for the week before her period.

Brianna began college that next fall with accommodations for her ADHD and OCD symptoms and continued to do well on her stimulant medication. She required a single dorm room, preferential registration to allow her to arrange her class schedule so that she could schedule classes when her medications were maximally effective, extended time on tests because of her slow reading rate and need to re-read, and notetakers for lecture classes. Her college disabilities office also offered coaching and help with transition to college.

CONCLUSION

Diagnosing ADHD is not a simple matter under the best of circumstances. Include coexisting conditions and gender issues and you add layers of complexity to this process. In addition, physiological factors may have a significant impact, not only on the diagnosis, but also on the choice of treatment regimens and outcomes for girls with ADHD. Parents and the professionals involved in the diagnostic process need to be aware of the additional burdens a girl with ADHD may be carrying. Societal and hormonal stressors need to be assessed and factored in when recommending a treatment program.

The use of medication in girls with ADHD may not be as simple as the choice of a stimulant, but may necessitate a more complex approach, one that uses therapies and medications in various combinations. And, in some instances, after careful consideration, parents may decide that medication is not the appropriate choice for their daughter with ADHD. In these circumstances, as in all cases of ADHD, it is critical that educators, mental health professionals, physicians, parents, and the girls themselves need to become more knowledgeable about the unique presentation of ADHD in girls and what can be done to help them.

CHAPTER TWELVE

Putting Our Understanding Into Action

AS WITH ALL GROUND-BREAKING topics in the study of human behavior, clinical practice often precedes research. The first edition of this book, published in 1999, was based on the many years of clinical experience that formed our understanding of girls with ADHD, and how they can be helped. At that time, this was the first and only book that focused exclusively on girls with ADHD. In the intervening years, an encouraging amount of research on girls and women has taken place. We hope that our insights and observations published in the first edition of *Understanding Girls with ADHD* was a catalyst to this much-needed research on girls with ADHD.

At the time of the publication of our first edition, the little research that existed on girls with ADHD narrowly focused on those few girls who met the male-based diagnostic guidelines laid out in the *Diagnostic and Statistical Manual, 4th Edition (DSM-IV)*[1] and earlier. As this book is written, the 5th edition of the DSM (DSM-5)[2] has recently been published, broadening the guidelines slightly, to include those that did not show clear signs of ADHD before the age of seven. As it is the hyperactive and behavior disordered children with ADHD (more likely to be boys) that are identified at an early age, this change in diagnostic criteria will certainly allow more girls to be correctly identified. Our continuing hope is that research will broaden over time to focus more on gender differences in those with ADHD.

One essential diagnostic question remains — how to develop and standardize gender appropriate criteria that can take into account the more subtle and internalized symptom patterns often found in girls. We also hope that the typical issues for girls with ADHD will be better defined, and that research will emerge that focuses on treatment modalities that best suit girls with ADHD. Today, most treatment programs for children with ADHD focus on problematic behaviors more typical of boys, and how to better control them in the classroom and at home. As we learn more about how to diagnose and treat girls, we hope that programs develop that can help girls with the self-esteem and relationship issues that are so challenging and damaging for them.

The earlier we learn to appropriately identify girls with ADHD, the less potential harm they will suffer. Even today, grown women are more likely to be diagnosed than young girls. A likely explanation that the sex ratios are almost equal in adults with ADHD is that women have the possibility of self-referral, whereas girls must rely on parents and teachers to refer them.

These women have waited half a lifetime for a diagnosis that can lead to understanding, self-acceptance, and success.

Because greater ADHD challenges for girls typically develop after puberty, perhaps the next wave of identification will take place in middle and high school. And, as the standard questionnaires used by teachers, parents, and pediatricians to identify young children are appropriately altered to include more female ADHD patterns, the wave will move down to elementary school-aged girls and to preschoolers. Those who are reading this revised edition of *Understanding Girls with ADHD* will join the growing ranks of parents and professionals working to bring about greater understanding of how best to diagnose and help girls with ADHD. While research on girls has increased significantly over the last few decades, it is still the case that the great majority of research continues to focus on predominantly male populations with relatively little research focused on the different patterns and issues found in girls with ADHD.

Early identification can help parents, teachers, and other professionals create environments to support and sustain these girls from their earliest years, helping them to feel strong, competent, and aware of their abilities. The more we learn, the more we are aware that the key to helping girls with ADHD is to create learning and working environments that suit their strengths.

Each girl with ADHD is unique. Those girls who are fortunate enough to be identified very early in life have a greater opportunity to benefit from the understanding and support of parents and educators that make appropriate choices for schooling, playmates, and play activities for them. What a difference it would make:

- If active, outgoing girls with ADHD had the good fortune to attend preschools that offered them more opportunity for movement, climbing, and socializing in active settings.

- If girls, who are quiet, disorganized daydreamers had the luxury of small group interaction and more individual attention from teachers.

- If creative girls with ADHD received more encouragement and validation for their artistic abilities and less discouragement for their messiness.

- If girls who are outspoken risk-takers were encouraged in sports or entrepreneurial activities rather than admonished for not being more well-behaved and lady-like.

While many boys with ADHD need help in controlling their impulses, reducing aggression, and becoming more compliant, many girls with ADHD need just the opposite. Daydreaming girls don't need help in learning to sit down and be quiet; they need lessons in how to stand up and advocate for themselves. They need to overcome their fears of asking for help, of raising their hand, and of answering the teacher's question incorrectly. More talkative, outgoing girls with ADHD need positive outlets for their social energy – permission and encouragement to take leadership positions in the classroom, to use their energy to plan and organize rather than to chatter disruptively. While many classroom guides for teachers emphasize the needs of boys with ADHD to move about, there is need for greater recognition of how to help girls, whose hyperactivity is often verbal, find appropriate, constructive verbal outlets.

For many girls with ADHD, their struggle is hidden — behind intense efforts to avoid notice, to please the teacher, and to get their work done. The brighter they are, the more easily they can hide their attentional difficulties, compensating with other strengths. Parents and professionals alike must be aware that young girls may successfully avoid overt difficulties for many years. It is a welcome change that the DSM-5, published in 2013, no longer requires that ADHD symptoms be evident before the age of seven in order to make a diagnosis. This single change makes it more likely that many girls that might have been overlooked through adherence to earlier criteria can now be appropriately identified and helped. The fact that some girls are quiet, obedient, above-average students makes their burgeoning ADHD no less real when it rears its head during adolescence with its many and greater challenges.

We are still on a learning curve in our understanding of girls with ADHD. We hope that parents who read this book will share it with professionals and teachers. Teachers should share it with counselors and school psychologists. Organizations and educational institutions need to sponsor more discussions and presentations on girls with ADHD. We all need to work together to raise the awareness of parents and professionals so that future generations of girls don't have to wait until they are women to finally receive a diagnosis that helps them to understand their differences, embrace their strengths, and finally live the life they deserve. It is our intention that this new edition of *Understanding Girls with ADHD* furthers that process.

APPENDIX

Self-Rating Scales Helping Identify Girls With ADHD

AS WE'VE WRITTEN ABOUT throughout this book, girls with ADHD are often overlooked and misunderstood. This questionnaire can be used to support girls by giving them a voice. We developed the following checklist to allow girls the opportunity to tell us about their internal experience of living with ADHD.

Most ADHD rating scales primarily focus upon observable behaviors as reported by others (parents and teachers). Because so many experiences of ADHD are internalized for girls, we can only become fully aware of the issues with which they struggle by asking them directly. This questionnaire is unique among ADHD questionnaires in offering girls an opportunity to directly self-report rather than relying upon parents and/or teachers to recognize their ADHD challenges.

This questionnaire was first developed in 1999, however, only recently has the importance of self-report questionnaires for girls with ADHD been recognized. In a 2013 study of gender differences[1] the most notable difference was greater anxiety in girls compared to boys. This anxiety was self-reported by girls, but not by their parents. Instead, parents mentioned somatic complaints, an outward manifestation of anxiety, without attributing these symptoms to anxiety. The authors of this study emphasize the importance of self-report scales in order to assess the internalizing problems that are especially salient in females with ADHD. We are very pleased that others in the ADHD field are starting to recognize the importance of self-report, particularly in studies exploring gender differences in ADHD.

This questionnaire is meant as a screening device, not a diagnostic tool. A girl's answers to this questionnaire should become prompts for further discussion. After this checklist is completed it should be reviewed with the girl by a parent, teacher or other professional. We find that reviewing responses to this questionnaire usually leads to a discussion of important issues that may not have been discussed before. This questionnaire gives girls a structured way that they can begin to express their feelings and to describe their struggles — the first step toward finding help and support for ADHD.

1. Skigli EW, Teicher MH, Andersen PN, Hovik KT & Oje M. (2013). ADHD in girls and boys – gender differences in coexisting symptoms and executive function measures. BMC *Psychiatry, 13*, 298.

ADHD Self-rating Scale for Girls

PATRICIA QUINN, M.D., KATHLEEN NADEAU, PH.D., AND ELLEN LITTMAN, PH.D.

Please respond to each item below rating it from 0 to 3 depending upon how well it describes you. Just do your best and try to rate each question as honestly as you can. There is no "right" or "wrong" answer. Your answers to these questions will allow the adults in your life to better understand and help you.

0 = Not at all like me
1 = A little like me
2 = Pretty much like me
3 = A lot like me

____ 1. I daydream a lot and can get lost in my own thoughts.
____ 2. No matter how hard I try, I often interrupt other people.
____ 3. When I'm upset, I say things that I don't mean.
____ 4. I feel restless inside when I have to sit or wait for a long time.
____ 5. I feel sleepy when I have to sit for a long time, but wake up and feel energetic as soon as I move around.
____ 6. I get frustrated because I am always losing things.
____ 7. I feel best when I'm active, such as playing sports, running, or dancing.
____ 8. My mind wanders when I'm trying to listen to the teacher.
____ 9. When I'm upset, I lose control and start yelling or screaming.
____ 10. Sometimes, I can get so excited that I start jumping around or talking loudly.
____ 11. I worry a lot.
____ 12. I'm scared to try new things because I don't think I can do them.
____ 13. I'm distracted by what other students are doing in class.
____ 14. It bothers me that I can't recall information I have just read or studied.
____ 15. I don't feel I'm as smart as other girls.
____ 16. I always seem to do or say the wrong thing when I'm around my friends.
____ 17. I feel like I'm not good at anything.
____ 18. I feel calmer after I exercise.
____ 19. I am very sensitive and my feelings get hurt a lot.
____ 20. I feel sad for no reason.
____ 21. Sometimes I feel so worried about school that I don't want to go.
____ 22. I often feel like I want to cry.
____ 23. I don't feel good about myself.

ADHD Self-rating Scale for Girls

PATRICIA QUINN, M.D., KATHLEEN NADEAU, PH.D., AND ELLEN LITTMAN, PH.D.

– continued –

____ 24. I feel embarrassed when people are watching me do something.
____ 25. I don't like to compete with other girls.
____ 26. I get nervous when I have to join a group, because I don't know what to say.
____ 27. I feel shy around my classmates.
____ 28. When other girls are laughing at something, I don't always get it.
____ 29. Sometimes a girl will walk away from me and I don't understand why.
____ 30. I wish I had more friends.
____ 31. I really try to be on time, even so, I'm still late for everything.
____ 32. I have trouble getting started on my homework.
____ 33. I feel like I'm "the problem kid" in my family.
____ 34. It's hard to fall asleep because my thoughts are racing in my brain.
____ 35. I hate myself and feel like a failure when I put things off until the last minute.
____ 36. I forget to do things.
____ 37. I feel people criticize me a lot.
____ 38. I have a difficult time getting up in the morning.
____ 39. I have trouble remembering the directions for an assignment.
____ 40. I like to do new things and feel bored doing the same old things.
____ 41. I spend a lot of time looking for things that I have misplaced.
____ 42. I feel bored a lot of the time.
____ 43. I get a lot of stomachaches or headaches.
____ 44. I like to do exciting, even scary, things.
____ 45. I often lose track of the time.
____ 46. I don't like to go into a crowded place.
____ 47. I'm often lost in class and feel everyone else knows what to do except me.
____ 48. Loud noises and/or bright lights bother me.
____ 49. I'm always worried that my teacher will be mad at me because I don't hear the directions, or can't answer a question when she calls on me.
____ 50. I have trouble making decisions.

Additional Questions for Teen Girls

PATRICIA QUINN, M.D., KATHLEEN NADEAU, PH.D., AND ELLEN LITTMAN, PH.D.

In addition to the previous 50 items, the following statements should be rated by girls 12-18 years. Please answer as honestly as you can using the same rating scale.

0 = Not at all like me
1 = A little like me
2 = Pretty much like me
3 = A lot like me

____ 1. It's hard for me to keep track of homework assignments and due dates.
____ 2. No matter how hard I try to be on time, I am usually late.
____ 3. I've convinced myself that I work best under pressure.
____ 4. I usually do assignments at the last minute, or turn assignments in late.
____ 5. High school feels overwhelming sometimes.
____ 6. People tell me that I need to try harder, but I feel like I'm doing the best I can.
____ 7. I sneak food and eat it when no one else is around.
____ 8. I start out each grading period determined to do well, but I can't keep it up for long.
____ 9. Sometimes when I am eating I just can't stop.
____ 10. I'm afraid of driving.
____ 11. My life feels frantic because I'm usually late or have forgotten something.
____ 12. It's hard for me to be patient.
____ 13. Sometimes I feel that I'm irresponsible.
____ 14. I jump from one topic to another in conversation.
____ 15. I don't always practice safe sex.
____ 16. I eat to calm myself down.
____ 17. I've had automobile accidents, or been stopped for speeding because I wasn't paying attention.
____ 18. I feel anxious pretty often.
____ 19. I use alcohol to help me feel better or forget about my problems.
____ 20. My moods and emotions are much more intense in the week before my period.

Additional Questions for Teen Girls

PATRICIA QUINN, M.D., KATHLEEN NADEAU, PH.D., AND ELLEN LITTMAN, PH.D.

– continued –

____ 21. I get frustrated very quickly.
____ 22. I make myself throw up or use laxatives to keep my weight in check.
____ 23. I feel moody and depressed, sometimes for no reason.
____ 24. I wish people understood how hard high school is for me and that I am really trying.
____ 25. Sometimes, I get angry and frustrated because of all the problems I have to face.
____ 26. I have hurt myself by cutting my arms or legs or pulling out my hair.
____ 27. I smoke cigarettes.
____ 28. I use marijuana.
____ 29. I have experimented with other drugs.
____ 30. I have trouble making and keeping friends.
____ 31. I have been the victim of bullying (including cyberbullying).
____ 32. I find that I overreact sometimes.
____ 33. I have thought about or tried to kill myself.
____ 34. My grades vary from A's to F's and I can't figure out why.
____ 35. I worry about doing well in college or even going to college.
____ 36. It bothers me that my grades seem to be getting worse as I get older.
____ 37. I need energy drinks, cola, or caffeine to stay awake.
____ 38. My mind gets mixed up and I have trouble saying what I want to say.
____ 39. I have difficulty standing up for myself or asking for help.
____ 40. I don't feel that I belong anywhere and feel alone

REFERENCES BY CHAPTER

INTRODUCTION

1. National Institutes of Health. (1994). NIH guidelines on the inclusion of women and minorities as subjects in clinical research. *NIH Guide, 23*, 1-34.
2. Hinshaw, S. P., Heller, T., & McHale, J. P. (1992). Covert antisocial behavior in boys with attention deficit hyperactivity disorder: External validation and effects of methylphenidate. *Journal of Consulting and Clinical Psychology, 60,* 274-281.
3. Hinshaw, S. P., Zupan, B. A., Simmel, C., Nigg, J. T., & Melnick, S. M. (1997). Peer status in boys with and without attention-deficit hyperactivity disorder: Predictions from overt and covert antisocial behavior, social isolation, and authoritative parenting beliefs. *Child Development, 64,* 880-896.
4. Arnold, L.E. (1996). Sex differences in ADHD: Conference summary. *Journal of Abnormal Child Psychology, 24*, 555-568.
5. Hinshaw, S. P. (2002). Preadolescent girls with attention-deficit/hyperactivity disorder: I. Background characteristics, comorbidity, cognitive and social functioning, and parenting practices. *Journal of Consulting and Clinical Psychology, 70*, 1086-1098.
6. Hinshaw, S. P., Carte, E. T., Sami, N., Treuting, J. J., & Zupan, B. A. (2002). Preadolescent girls with attention-deficit/hyperactivity disorder: II. Neuropsychological performance in relation to subtypes and individual classification. *Journal of Consulting and Clinical Psychology, 70*, 1099-1111.
7. Blachman, D. R., & Hinshaw, S. P. (2002). Patterns of friendship in girls with and without attention-deficit/hyperactivity disorder. *Journal of Abnormal Child Psychology, 30*, 625-640.
8. Briscoe-Smith, A. M., and Hinshaw, S. P. (2006). Linkages between child abuse and attention-deficit/hyperactivity disorder in girls: Behavioral and social correlates. *Child abuse and neglect, 30,* 1239-1255.
9. Mikami, A. Y., & Hinshaw, S. P. (2003). Buffers of peer rejection among girls with and without ADHD: The role of popularity with adults and goal-directed solitary play. *Journal of Abnormal Child Psychology, 31*, 381-397.

10. Peris, T., & Hinshaw, S. P. (2003). Family dynamics and preadolescent girls with ADHD: The relationship between expressed emotion, ADHD symptomatology, and comorbid disruptive behavior. *Journal of Child Psychology and Psychiatry, 44*, 1177-1190.
11. Sami, N., Carte, E. T., Hinshaw, S. P., & Zupan, B. A. (2003). Performance of girls with attention deficit/hyperactivity disorder on the Rey-Osterrieth Complex Figure: Evidence for executive function deficits. *Child Neuropsychology, 9*, 237-254.
12. Zalecki, C., & Hinshaw, S. P. (2004). Overt and relational aggression in girls with attention-deficit hyperactivity disorder. *Journal of Clinical Child and Adolescent Psychology, 33*, 131-143.
13. Gaub, M., & Carlson, C. L. (1997). Gender differences in ADHD: A meta-analysis and critical review. *Journal of the American Academy of Child and Adolescent Psychiatry, 36*, 1036-1046.
14. Gershon, J. (2002). A meta-analytic review of gender differences in ADHD. *Journal of Attention Disorders, 5*, 143-154.
15. Biederman, J., Faraone, S. V., Mick, E., Williamson, S., Wilens, T., Spencer, T. J., et al. (1999). Clinical correlates of ADHD in females: Findings from a large group of girls ascertained from pediatric and psychiatric referral sources. *Journal of the American Academy of Child and Adolescent Psychiatry, 38*, 966-975.
16. Hinshaw, S. P., Owens, E. B., Sami, N., & Fargeon, S. (2006). Prospective follow-up of girls with attention-deficit/hyperactivity disorder into adolescence: Evidence for continuing cross-domain impairment. *Journal of Consulting and Clinical Psychology, 74*, 489-499.
17. Hinshaw, S. P., Carte, E. T., Fan, C., Jassy, J. S., & Owens, E. B. (2007). Neuropsychological functioning of girls with attention-deficit/hyperactivity disorder followed prospectively into adolescence: Evidence for continuing deficits? *Neuropsychology, 21*, 263-273.
18. Hinshaw, S., Owens, E., Zalecki, C., Huggins, S., Montenegro-Nevado, A., Schrodek, E., & Swanson, E. (2012). Prospective follow-up of girls with attention-deficit/hyperactivity disorder into early adulthood: Continuing impairment includes elevated risk for suicide attempts and self-injury. *Journal of Consulting and Clinical Psychology, 80*, 1041-1051.
19. Biederman, J., Petty, C.R., Monuteaux, M.C., Fried, R., Byrne, D., Mirto, T., et al. (2010). Adult psychiatric outcomes of girls with attention deficit hyperactivity disorder: 11-year follow-up in a longitudinal case-control study. *American Journal of Psychiatry, 167*, 409–417.
20. Hinshaw, S. P., Owens, E. B., Sami, N., & Fargeon, S. (2006). Prospective follow-up of girls with attention-deficit/hyperactivity disorder into adolescence: Evidence for continuing cross-domain impairment. *Journal of Consulting and Clinical Psychology, 74*, 489-499.
21. Hinshaw, S. P., Carte, E. T., Fan, C., Jassy, J. S., & Owens, E. B. (2007). Neuropsychological functioning of girls with attention-deficit/hyperactivity disorder followed prospectively into adolescence: Evidence for continuing deficits? *Neuropsychology, 21*, 263-273.
22. Owens, E. B., Hinshaw, S. P., Lee, S. S., & Lahey, B. B. (2009). Few girls with childhood attention-deficit/hyperactivity disorder show positive adjustment during adolescence. *Journal of Clinical Child and Adolescent Psychology, 38*, 1-12.
23. Miller, M., Ho, J., & Hinshaw, S. P. (2012). Executive functions in girls with ADHD followed prospectively into young adulthood. *Neuropsychology, 26*, 278-287.
24. Miller, M., Montenegro-Nevado, A. J., & Hinshaw, S. P. (2012). Childhood executive function continues to predict outcomes in young adult females with and without childhood diagnosed ADHD. *Journal of Abnormal Child Psychology, 40*, 657-668.
25. Hinshaw, S., Owens, E., Zalecki, C., Huggins, S., Montenegro-Nevado, A., Schrodek, E., & Swanson, E. (2012). Prospective follow-up of girls with attention-deficit/hyperactivity disorder into early adulthood: Continuing impairment includes elevated risk for suicide attempts and self-injury. *Journal of Consulting and Clinical Psychology, 80*, 1041-1051.

26. Swanson, E. N., Owens, E. B., & Hinshaw, S. P. (2014). Pathways to self-harmful behaviors in young women with and without ADHD: A longitudinal investigation of mediating factors. *Journal of Child Psychology and Psychiatry, 44*, 505-515.
27. Chronis-Tuscano, A., Molina, B. S. G., Pelham, W. E, Applegate, B., Dahlke, A., Overmeyer, M., & Lahey, B. B. (2010). Very early predictors of adolescent depression and suicide attempts in children with attention-deficit/hyperactivity disorder. *Archives of General Psychiatry, 67*, 1044-1051.
28. Hinshaw, S. P., with Kranz, R. (2009). *The triple bind: Saving our teenage girls from today's pressures*. New York: Random House/Ballantine.
29. Swanson, E. N., Owens, E. B., & Hinshaw, S. P. (2014). Pathways to self-harmful behaviors in young women with and without ADHD: A longitudinal investigation of mediating factors. *Journal of Child Psychology and Psychiatry, 44*, 505-515.
30. Guendelman, M., Owens, E. B., Galan, C., Gard, A., & Hinshaw, S. P. (2014). Early-adult correlates of maltreatment in girls with ADHD: Increased risk for internalizing symptoms and suicidality. Manuscript submitted for publication.
31. Hinshaw, S. P., & Scheffler, R. M. (2014). *The ADHD explosion: Myths, medication, money, and today's push for performance*. New York: Oxford University Press.
32. Hinshaw, S. P. (2013). Developmental psychopathology as a scientific discipline: Rationale, principles, and recent advances. In T. P. Beauchaine & S. P. Hinshaw (Eds.), *Child and adolescent psychopathology* (2nd ed., pp. 1-18). Hoboken, NJ: Wiley.
33. Hinshaw, S. P. (2007). *The mark of shame: Stigma of mental illness and an agenda for change*. New York: Oxford University Press.

CHAPTER ONE

1. Abikoff, H., Courtney, M. E., Pelham, W. E., Jr., & Koplewicz, H. S. (1993). Teachers' ratings of disruptive behaviors: The influence of halo effects. *Journal of Abnormal Child Psychology, 21*, 519–533.
2. Ohan, J., & Visser, T. (2009). Why is there a gender gap in children presenting for attention deficit/hyperactivity disorder services? *Journal of Clinical Child and Adolescent Psychology, 38*, 650-660.
3. Derks, E. M., Hudziak, J. J., & Boomsma, D. I. (2007). Why more boys than girls with ADHD receive treatment: A study of Dutch twins. *Twin Research and Human Genetics, 10(5)*, 765-770. doi:10.1375/twin.10.5.765.
4. American Psychiatric Association. (2013). *Diagnostic and statistical manual of mental disorders, Fifth edition*. Arlington, VA: American Psychiatric Publishers.
5. Almagor, D. (2011). Gender differences and age of diagnosis in ADHD. *Abnormal Child Psychology, 21*, 519–533.
6. Simon, V., Czobor, P., Balint, S., Meszaros, A., & Bitter, I. (2009). Prevalence and correlates of adult attention deficit hyperactivity disorder: Meta-analysis. *The British Journal of Psychiatry*, (2009) 194, 204–211. doi: 10.1192/bjp.bp.107.048827
7. American Psychiatric Association. (2013). *Diagnostic and statistical manual of mental disorders, Fifth edition*. Arlington, VA: American Psychiatric Publishers.
8. Brown, T. (1996, 2001) *Brown Attention-Deficit Scales (Brown ADD Scales)*. San Antonio, TX: Pearson.
9. Biederman, J., Faraone, S.V., Spencer, T., Wilens, T., Norman, D., Lapey, K.A., Mick, E., Lehman, B.K., & Doyle, A. (1993). Patterns of psychiatric comorbidity, cognition, and psychosocial functioning in adults with attention deficit/ hyperactivity disorder. *American Journal of Psychiatry, 150*(12), 1792-1798.
10. Ohan, J. L., & Johnston, C. (2005). Gender appropriateness of symptom criteria for attention-deficit/hyperactivity disorder, oppositional defiant disorder, and conduct Disorder. *Child Psychiatry and Human Development, 35*, 359-381.

11. Biederman, J., Faraone, S., Mick, E., et al. (1999). Clinical correlates of ADHD in females: Findings from a large group of girls ascertained from pediatric and psychiatric referral services. *Journal of the American Academy of Child and Adolescent Psychiatry, 38* (8), 966-975.
12. Arnold, L.E. (1996.) Sex differences in ADHD: Conference summary. *Journal of Abnormal Child Psychology, 24* (5), 555-568.
13. O'Brien, J., Dowell, L., Mostofsky, S., Denckla, M., & Mahone, E.M. (2010). Neuropsychological profiles of executive function in girls with attention-deficit/hyperactivity disorder. *Archives of Clinical Neuropsychology, 25*(7): 656–670.
14. Arnold, L.E. (1996). Sex differences in ADHD: Conference summary. *Journal of Abnormal Child Psychology, 24* (5), 555-568.
15. Ohan, J. L., & Johnston, C. (2007). What is the social impact of ADHD in girls? A multi-method assessment. *Journal of Abnormal Child Psychology, 35*(2), 239-250.
16. Gaub, M., & Carlson, C. (1997). Gender differences in ADHD: A meta-analysis and critical review. *Journal of the American Academy of Child and Adolescent Psychiatry, 36* (8), 1036-1045.
17. Gaub, M., & Carlson, C. (1997). Gender differences in ADHD: A meta-analysis and critical review. *Journal of the American Academy of Child and Adolescent Psychiatry, 36* (8), 1036-1045.
18. Brown, R., Madau-Swain, A., & Baldwin, K. (1991). Gender differences in a clinic-referred sample of attention deficit disordered children. *Child Psychiatry and Human Development, 22*, 111-128.
19. Silverthorn, P. (1996). Developing a model for explaining antisocial behavior in girls. The University of Alabama, ProQuest, UMI Dissertations Publishing, 1996. 9808257
20. Blachman, D.R., & Hinshaw, S.P. (2002). Patterns of friendship among girls with and without attention-deficit/hyperactivity disorder. *Journal of Abnormal Child Psychology, 30* (6), 625-640.
21. Johnson, J., McCown, W., & Booker, M. (1986). *MMPI profiles of multiply-abused and sheltered women*. Paper presented at the meeting of the Midwestern Psychological Association, Chicago, IL.
22. Arcia, E., & Conners, C.K. (1998). Gender differences in ADHD? *Journal of Developmental and Behavioral Pediatrics, 19* (2), 77-83.
23. Rucklidge, J., & Tannock, R. (2001). Psychiatric, psychosocial and cognitive functioning of female adolescents with ADHD. *Journal of the American Academy of Child and Adolescent Psychiatry, 40*(5); 530-540.
24. Huessy, H.R. (1990). *The pharmacotherapy of personality disorders in women*. Paper presented at the annual meeting of the American Psychiatric Association (symposia), New York.
25. Biederman, J., Monuteaux, M.C., Mick, E., et al. (2006). Psychopathology in females with attention-deficit/hyperactivity ddisorder: A controlled, five-year prospective study. *Biological Psychiatry, 60*, 1098–1105.
26. Owens, E.B., Hinshaw, S.P., Lee, L.L., & Lahey, B.B. (2009). Few girls with children ADHD show positive adjustment during adolescence. *Journal of Clinical Child and Adolescent Psychology, 38*, 132-143.
27. Rucklidge, J.J., & Tannock, R. (2001). Psychiatric, psychosocial, and cognitive functioning of female adolescents with AD/HD. *Journal of the American Academy of Child and Adolescent Psychiatry, 40*, 530-540.
28. Dalsgaard, S., Mortensen, P.B., Frydenberg, M., & Thomsen, P.H. (2002). Conduct problems, gender and adult psychiatric outcome of children with attention-deficit hyperactivity disorder. *British Journal of Psychiatry, 181*, 416-421.
29. Hinshaw, S.P., Owens, E.B., Zalecki, C., Huggins, S.P. et al. (2012). Prospective follow-up of girls with attention-deficit/hyperactivity disorder into early adulthood: Continuing

impairment includes elevated risk for suicide attempts and self-injury. *Journal Consulting and Clinical Psychology, 80,* 1041-51.
30. Mikami, A., & Hinshaw, S. (2006). Resilient adolescent adjustment among girls: buffers of childhood peer rejection and attention-deficit/hyperactivity disorder. *Journal of Abnormal Child Psychology, 34,* 825-839.
31. Biederman, J., Milberger, S., Faraone, S., Kiely, K., Guite, J., Mick, E., Ablon, S., Warburton, R., Reed, E., & Davis, S. (1995). Impact of adversity on functioning and comorbidity in children with attention-deficit hyperactivity disorder. *Journal of the American Academy of Child and Adolescent Psychiatry, 34* (11), 1495-1503.

CHAPTER TWO

1. Barkley, R. A. (1997). Attention-deficit/hyperactivity disorder, self-regulation, and time: Toward a more comprehensive theory. *Journal of Developmental and Behavioral Pediatrics, 18,* 271–279.
2. Willcutt, E.G., Doyle, A.E., Nigg, J.T., Faraone, S.V., & Pennington, B.F. (2005). Validity of the executive function theory of attention-deficit/hyperactivity disorder: A meta-analytic review. *Biological Psychiatry, 57,* 1–1346.
3. American Psychiatric Association. (2013). *Diagnostic and statistical manual of mental disorders, Fifth edition.* Washington, DC.
4. Arnsten, A.F. (2009). The emerging neurobiology of attention deficit hyperactivity disorder: The key role of the prefrontal association cortex. *Journal of Pediatrics, 154,* S1-S43.
5. Barkley, R. (2000). *Taking charge of ADHD. The complete, authoritative guide for parents.* New York, NY: Guilford Press.
6. Goldstein, S. (1999). Attention-deficit/hyperactivity disorder. In S. Goldstein & C. R. Reynolds (Eds.), *Handbook of neurodevelopmental and genetic disorders in children* (pp. 154–175) New York, NY: Guilford Press.
7. Nigg, J. (2006). *What causes ADHD?: Understanding what goes wrong and why.* New York, NY: Guilford Press.
8. Harris, M.N., Voigt, R.G., Barbaresi, W.J., Voge, G.A., Killian, J.M., Weaver, A.L., Colby, C.E., Carey, W.A., & Katusic, S.K. (2013). ADHD and learning disabilities in former late preterm infants: A population-based birth cohort. *Pediatrics, 132,* e630-636.
9. Faraone, S.V., Perlis, R.H., Doyle, A.E., et al. (2005). Molecular genetics of attention deficit hyperactivity disorder. *Biological Psychiatry, 57,* 1-1.
10. Biederman, J., Faraone, S.V., Mick, E., Spencer, T., Wilens, T., Kieley, K., et al. (1995). High risk for attention deficit hyperactivity disorder among children of parents with childhood onset of the disorder: A pilot study. *American Journal of Psychiatry, 152,* 431-435.
11. Arnsten, A.F.T., & Rubia, K. (2012). Neurobiological circuits regulating attention, cognitive control, motivation, and emotion: Disruptions in neurodevelopmental psychiatric disorders. *Journal of the American Academy of Child and Adolescent Psychiatry, 51,* 356-367.
12. Castellanos, F.X., Lee, P.P., Sharp, W., et al. (2002). Developmental trajectories of brain volume abnormalities in children and adolescents with attention-deficit/hyperactivity disorder. *Journal of the American Medical Association, 288,* 1740-1748.
13. Shaw, P., Lerch, J., Greenstein, D., Sharp, W., et al., (2006). Longitudinal mapping of cortical thickness and clinical outcome in children and adolescents with attention deficit/hyperactivity disorder. *Archives of General Psychiatry, 63,* 540-549.
14. Shaw, P., Eckstrand, K., Sharp, W., Blumenthal, J., Lerch, J.P., et. al., (2007). Attention-deficit/hyperactivity disorder is characterized by a delay in cortical maturation. *Proceedings of the National Academy of Science, 104,* 19649-19654.
15. Shaw, P., & Rabin, C. (2009). New insights into attention-deficit/hyperactivity disorder using structural neuroimaging. *Current Psychiatry Reports, 11,* 393-398.

16. Makris, N., Biederman, J., Valera, E.M., et al. (2007). Cortical thinning of the attention and executive function networks in adults with attention-deficit/hyperactivity disorder. *Cerebral Cortex, 17*, 1364-1375.
17. Arnsten, A.F. (2009). Toward a new understanding of attention-deficit hyperactivity disorder pathophysiology: An important role for prefrontal cortex dysfunction. *CNS Drugs, 23*, 33-41.
18. Bush, G. (2010). Attention-deficit/hyperactivity disorder and attention networks. *Neuropsychopharmacologic Review, 35*, 278-300.
19. Hynd, G., Segmund-Clieman, M., Lorys, A.R., Novey, D., & Eliopulos, D. (1990). Brain morphology in developmental dyslexia and attention deficit hyperactivity disorder. *Archives of Neurology, 47*, 919-926.
20. Hynd, G., Segmund-Clieman, M., Lorys, A.R., Novey, D., Eliopulos, D., & Lyytinen, H. (1991). Corpus callosum morphology in attention deficit hyperactivity disorder: Morphometric analysis of MRI. *Journal of Learning Disabilities, 24*, 141-146.
21. Mattfeld, A.T., Gabrieli, J.D., Biederman, J., Spencer, T., Brown, A., Kotte, A., Kagan, E., & Whitfield-Gabrieli, S. (2014). Brain differences between persistent and remitted attention deficit hyperactivity disorder. *Brain, 37,* 2423-2428
22. Filipek, P.A., Segmund-Clieman, M., Steingard, R.J., et al. (1997). Volumetric MRI analysis comparing subjects having attention deficit hyperactivity disorder with normal controls. *Neurology, 48*, 587-601.
23. Castellanos, F.X., Giedd, J.N., Marsh, W.L., et al. (1996). Quantitative brain magnetic resonance imaging in attention-deficit hyperactivity disorder. *Archives of General Psychiatry, 53*, 607-616.
24. Arnsten, A.F. (2009). Toward a new understanding of attention-deficit hyperactivity disorder pathophysiology: An important role for prefrontal cortex dysfunction. *CNS Drugs, 23,* (suppl 1), 33-41.
25. Mahone, E.M., Crocetti, D., Ranta, M.E., Gaddis, A., Cataldo, M., Slifer, K.J., Denckla, M.B., & Mostofsky, S.H. (2011). A preliminary neuroimaging study of preschool children with ADHD. *The Clinical Neuropsychologist, 25*, 1009-1028.
26. Arnsten, A.F.T., & Rubia, K. (2012). Neurobiological circuits regulating attention, cognitive control, motivation, and emotion: Disruptions in neurodevelopmental psychiatric disorders. *Journal of the American Academy of Child and Adolescent Psychiatry, 51,* 356-367.
27. Miyake, A., Friedman, N.P., Emerson, M.J., Witzki, A.H., et al. (2000). Unity and diversity of executive functions and their contribution to complex 'frontal lobe' tasks: A latent variable analysis. *Cognitive Psychology, 41*, 49-100.
28. Caviness, V.S., Kennedy, D.N., Richelme, C., et al. (1996). The human brain age 7-11 years: A volumetric analysis based on magnetic resonance images. *Cerebral Cortex, 6,* 726-736.
29. Anderson, S.L., Rutstein, M., Benzo, J.M., et al. (1997). Sex differences in dopamine receptor overproduction and elimination. *NeuroReport, 8,* 1495-1498.
30. McEwen, B.S., Alves, S.E., Bullock, K., & Weiland, N.G. (1997). Ovarian steroids and the brain: Implications for cognition and aging. *Neurology, 48*, Supplement, 8-15.
31. Fink, G., Sumner, B.E., Rosie, R., Grace, O., & Quinn, J.P. (1996). Estrogen control of central neurotransmission: Effect on mood, mental state, and memory. *Cell Molecular Biology, 16*, -344.
32. Huessy, H. R. (1990). The pharmacotherapy of personality disorders in women. Paper presented at the annual meeting of the American Psychiatric Association (symposia), New York.
33. Dorn, L. D., Hitt, S.F., & Rotenstein, D. (1999). Biopsychological and cognitive differences in children with premature vs. on-time adrenarche. *Archives of Pediatric and Adolescent Medicine, 153*, 137-146.

34. Sheridan, M.A., Hinshaw, S., & Esposito, M. (2007). Efficiency of the prefrontal cortex during working memory in attention-deficit/hyperactivity disorder. *Journal of the American Academy of Child and Adolescent Psychiatry, 46*, 1357-1366.
35. Seidman, L.J., Biederman. J., Faraone, S.V., Weber. W., Mennin. D., & Jones, J. (1997). A pilot study of neuropsychological function in girls with ADHD. *Journal of the American Academy of Child and Adolescent Psychiatry, 36*, 366-373.
36. Ernst, M., Liebenauer, L.L., King, A., et al. (1994). Reduced brain metabolism in hyperactive girls. *Journal of the American Academy of Child and Adolescent Psychiatry, 33*, 858-868.

CHAPTER THREE

1. Hardy, K.K., Kollins, S.H., Murray, D.W., Riddle, M.A., Greenhill, L., et al. (2007). Factor structure of parent- and teacher-rated symptoms in the preschoolers with attention-deficit/hyperactivity disorder treatment study (PATS). *Journal of Child and Adolescent Psychopharmacology, 17*, 621-634.
2. Law, E.C., Sideridis, G.D., Prock, L.A., & Sheridan, M.A. (2014). Attention-deficit/hyperactivity disorder in young children: Predictors of diagnostic stability. *Pediatrics, 133*, 659-667.
3. Lee, S.S., Lahey, B.B., Owens, B.B. & Hinshaw, S.P. (2008). Few preschool boys and girls with ADHD are well-adjusted during adolescence. *Journal of Abnormal Child Psychology, 36*, 373-383.
4. AAP, SUBCOMMITTEE ON ATTENTION-DEFICIT/HYPERACTIVITY DISORDER, STEERING COMMITTEE ON QUALITY IMPROVEMENT AND MANAGEMENT (2011) ADHD: Clinical practice guideline for the diagnosis, evaluation, and treatment of attention-deficit/hyperactivity disorder in children and adolescents. *Pediatrics, 128*, 2011-2654.
5. Curchack-Lichtin, J.T., Chacko, A., & Halperin, J.M. (2013). Changes in ADHD symptom endorsement: Preschool to school age. *Journal of Abnormal Child Psychology, 42*, 993-1004.
6. Byrne, J.M., Bawden, H.N., Beattie, T.L., DeWolfe, N.A. (2000). Preschoolers classified as having attention-deficit hyperactivity disorder (ADHD): DSM-IV symptom endorsement pattern. *Journal of Child Neurology, 15*, 533-538.
7. Wilens, T.E., Biederman, J., Brown, S., Monuteaux, M., Prince, J., & Spencer, T.J. (2002). Patterns of psychopathology and dysfunction in clinically referred preschoolers. *Journal of Developmental and Behavioral Pediatrics, 23*, S31-36.
8. Wilens, T.E., Biederman, J., Brown, S., Tanguay, S., Monuteaux, M.C., Blake, C., & Spencer, T.J. (2002). Psychiatric comorbidity and functioning in clinically referred preschool children and school-aged youth with ADHD. *Journal of the American Academy of Child and Adolescent Psychiatry, 41*, 262-268.
9. Nichamin, S. (1972). Recognizing minimal cerebral dysfunction in the infant and toddler. *Clinical Pediatrics, 11*, 255-257.
10. Matheny, A.P., Brown, A.M., & Wilson, R.S. (1971). Behavioral antecedents of accidental injuries in early childhood: A study of twins. *Journal of Pediatrics, 79*, 122-124.
11. Matheny, A.P., Brown, A.M., & Wilson, R.S. (1972). Assessment of children's behavioral characteristics: A toll in accident prevention. *Clinical Pediatrics, 11*, 437-439.
12. Miller, C.J., Miller, S.R,, Healey, D.M., Marshall, K., & Halperin, J.M. (2013). Are cognitive control and stimulus-driven processes differentially linked to inattention and hyperactivity in preschoolers? *Journal of Clinical Child and Adolescent Psychology, 42*, 187-196.
13. Dadgarnia, M.H., Baradaranfar, M.H., Fallah, R., Atighechi, S., et al. (2012). Effect of adenotonsillectomy on ADHD symptoms of children with adenotonsillar hypertrophy. *Acta Medica Iran, 50*, 547-551.

14. American Psychiatric Association. (2013). *Diagnostic and statistical manual of mental disorders, Fifth edition.* Arlington, VA: American Psychiatric Association.
15. Waldrop, M., Bell, R., McLaughlin, B., et al. (1978). Newborn minor physical anomalies predict short attention span, peer aggression, and impulsivity at age 3. *Science, 199*, 563-565.
16. Montes, G., Lotyczewski, B.S., Halterman, J.S., & Hightower, A.D. (2012). School readiness among children with behavior problems at entrance into kindergarten: Results from a US national study. *European Journal of Pediatrics, 171*, 541-548.
17. Miller, C.J., Miller, S.R., Healey, D.M., Marshall, K., & Halperin, J.M. (2013). Are cognitive control and stimulus-driven processes differentially linked to inattention and hyperactivity in preschoolers? *Journal of Clinical Child and Adolescent Psychology, 42*, 187-96.
18. Richman, N., Stevenson, J.E., & Graham, P.J. (1975). Prevalence of behavior problems in 3-year-old children: An epidemiological study in a London borough. *Journal of Child Psychology and Psychiatry, 16*, 277-287.
19. Coleman, J., Wolkind, S., & Ashley, L. (1977). Symptoms of behavior disturbance and adjustment to school. *Journal of Child Psychology and Psychiatry, 18*, 201-209.
20. Petersen, I.T., Bates, J.E., D'Onofrio, B.M., Coyne, C.A., Lansford, J.E., Dodge, K.A., Pettit, G.S., & Van Hulle, C.A. (2013). Language ability predicts the development of behavior problems in children. *Journal of Abnormal Psychology, 122*, 542-557.
21. Rohrer-Baumgartner, N., Zeiner, P., Eadie, P., Egeland, J., Gustavson, K,, Reichborn-Kjennerud, T., & Aase, H. (2013). Language delay in 3-year-old children with ADHD Symptoms. *Journal of Attention Disorders*, Aug 13. [Epub ahead of print]
22. Spira, E.G., & Fischel, J.E. (2005) The impact of preschool inattention, hyperactivity, and impulsivity on social and academic development: A review. *Journal of Child Psychology and Psychiatry, 46*, 755-773.
23. Sims, D.M., & Lonigan, C.J. (2013). Inattention, hyperactivity, and emergent literacy: Different facets of inattention relate uniquely to preschoolers' reading-related skills. *Journal of Clinical Child and Adolescent Psychology, 42*, 208-219.
24. Sáez, L., Folsom, J.S., Al Otaiba, S., & Schatschneider, C. (2012). Relations among student attention behaviors, teacher practices, and beginning word reading skill. *Journal of Learning Disabilities, 45*, 418-432.
25. Schoemaker, K., Bunte, T., Espy, K.A., Deković, M.,& Matthys, W. (2014). Executive functions in preschool children with ADHD and DBD: An 18-month longitudinal study. *Developmental Neuropsychology, 39*, 302-.
26. Korsch, F., & Petermann, F. (2014). Agreement between parents and teachers on preschool children's behavior in a clinical sample with externalizing behavioral problems. *Child Psychiatry and Human Development, 45*, 617-627.
27. Tripp, G., Schaughency, E.A., & Clarke, B. (2006). Parent and teacher rating scales in the evaluation of attention-deficit hyperactivity disorder: Contribution to diagnosis and differential diagnosis in clinically referred children. *Journal of Developmental and Behavioral Pediatrics, 27*, 209-218.
28. Biederman, J., Faraone, S.V., Mick, E., Spencer, T., Wilens, T., Kieley, K., et al. (1995). High risk for attention deficit hyperactivity disorder among children of parents with childhood onset of the disorder: A pilot study. *American Journal of Psychiatry, 152*, 431-435.
29. Charach, A., Carson, P., Fox, S., Ali, M.U., Beckett, J., & Lim, C.G. (2013). Interventions for preschool children at high risk for ADHD: A comparative effectiveness review. *Pediatrics, 131*, e1584-1604.
30. Charach, A., Carson, P., Fox, S., Ali, M.U., Beckett, J., & Lim, C.G. (2013). Interventions for preschool children at high risk for ADHD: A comparative effectiveness review. *Pediatrics, 131*, e1584-1604.

31. Herbert, S.D., Harvey, E.A., Roberts, J.L., Wichowski, K., & Lugo-Candelas, C.I. (2012). A randomized controlled trial of a parent training and emotion socialization program for families of hyperactive preschool-aged children. *Behavior Therapy, 44*, 302-.
32. Greenhill, L., Kollins, S., Abikoff, H., McCracken, J., Riddle, M., et al. (2006). Efficacy and safety of immediate-release methylphenidate treatment for preschoolers with ADHD. *Journal of the American Academy of Child and Adolescent Psychiatry, 45*, 1284-1293.
33. Halperin, J.M., Marks, D.J., Bedard, A.C., Chacko, A., Curchach, J.T., Yoon, C.A., & Healey, D.M. (2013). Training executive, attention, and motor skills: A proof-of-concept study in preschool children with ADHD. *Journal of Attention Disorders, 17*, 711-721.

CHAPTER FOUR

1. Best, J., & Miller, P. (2010). A developmental perspective on executive function. *Child Development, 81*, 1641–1660.
2. Piaget, J. (1929). *The child's conception of the world.* London: Routledge and Kegan Paul.
3. Maccoby, E. (1998). *The two sexes: Growing up apart, coming together.* Cambridge, MA: Belknap-Harvard University Press.
4. Gaub, M., & Carlson, C. (1997). Gender differences in ADHD: A meta-analysis and critical review. *Journal of the American Academy of Child and Adolescent Psychiatry, 36*, 1036-1045.
5. Henker, B., & Whalen, C. (1999). The child with attention-deficit/hyperactivity disorder in school and peer settings. In C. Quay & A. Hogan (eds), *Handbook of Disruptive Behavior Disorders.* (pp157-178). New York, NY: Kluwer Academic/Plenum.
6. American Psychiatric Association (2013). *Diagnostic and statistical manual of mental disorders, Fifth edition.* American Psychiatric Association: Washington DC.
7. Nigg, J., Tannock, R., & Rohde, L. (2010). What is to be the fate of ADHD subtypes? An introduction to the special section on research on the ADHD subtypes and implications for the DSM-5. *Journal of Clinical Child and Adolescent Psychology, 39*, 723-725.
8. Elkins, I., Malone, S., Keyes, M., Iacono, W., & McGue, M. (2011). The impact of attention-deficit/hyperactivity disorder on preadolescent adjustment may be greater for girls than for boys. *Journal of Clinical Child and Adolescent Psychology, 40*, 532-545.
9. Fontaine, N., Carbonneau, R., Barker, E., Vitaro, F., Hebert, M., Cote, S., Nagin, D., Zoccolillo, M., & Tremblay, R. (2008). Girls' hyperactivity and physical aggression during childhood and adjustment problems in early adulthood: A 15-year longitudinal study. *Archives of General Psychiatry, 65*, -.
10. Faraone, S., Biederman J., & Mick, E. (2006a). The age-dependent decline of attention deficit hyperactivity disorder: A meta-analysis of follow-up studies. *Psychological Medicine, 36*, 159–165.
11. Hinshaw, S., Owens, L., Sami, N., & Fargeon, S. (2006). Prospective follow-up of girls with attention-deficit/hyperactivity disorder are independent of oppositional defiant or reading disorder. *Journal of the American Academy of Child and Adolescent Psychiatry, 20*, 209-216.
12. Counts, C., Nigg, J., Stawicki, J., Rappley, M., & Von Eye, A. (2005). Family adversity in DSM-IV ADHD combined and inattentive subtypes and associated disruptive behavior problems. *Journal of the American Academy of Child and Adolescent Psychiatry, 44*, 690–698.
13. Biederman, J., Mick, E., Faraone, S., Braaten, E., Doyle, A., Spencer, T., et al. (2002). Influence of gender on attention deficit hyperactivity disorder in children referred to a psychiatric clinic. *American Journal of Psychiatry, 159*, 36-42.
14. Elkins, I., Malone, S., Keyes, M., Iacono, W., & McGue, M. (2011). The impact of attention-deficit/hyperactivity disorder on preadolescent adjustment may be greater for girls than for boys. *Journal of Clinical Child and Adolescent Psychology, 40*, 532-545.

15. Elkins, I., Malone, S., Keyes, M., Iacono, W., & McGue, M. (2011). The impact of attention-deficit/hyperactivity disorder on preadolescent adjustment may be greater for girls than for boys. *Journal of Clinical Child and Adolescent Psychology, 40*, 532-545.
16. Hinshaw, S. (2002). Preadolescent girls with attention-deficit/hyperactivity disorder: I. Background characteristics, comorbidity, cognitive and social functioning, and parenting practices. *Journal of Consulting and Clinical Psychology, 70*, 1086-1098.
17. Staller, J., & Faraone, S. (2006). Attention deficit hyperactivity disorders in girls: Epidemiology and management. *CNS Drugs, 20*, 170-173.
18. Bauermeister, J. (2007). ADHD and gender: Are risks and sequela of ADHD the same for boys and girls? *Journal of Child Psychology and Psychiatry, 48*, 831-839.
19. Kaufmann, F., & Castellanos, X. (2000). Attention-deficit/hyperactivity disorder in gifted students. In K. Heller, F. Monks, R. Sternberg. & R. Subotnik (eds) *International handbook of giftedness and talent, 2nd ed.*, 621-632. Amsterdam:Elsevier.
20. Chae, P.K., Kim, J.H., & Noh K.S. (2003). Diagnosis of ADHD among gifted children in relation to KEDI-WISC and T.O.V.A. performance. *Gifted Child Quarterly, 47*, 192-201.
21. Barkley, R. (1998). *Attention deficit hyperactivity disorder: A handbook for diagnosis and treatment.* New York, NY: Guilford Press.
22. Leroux, J., & Levitt-Perlman, M. (2000). The gifted child with attention deficit disorder: An identification and intervention challenge. *Roeper Review, 22,* 171-176.
23. Antshel, K., Faraone, S., Maglione, K., Doyle, A., Fried, R., Seidman, L., & Biederman, J. (2008). Temporal stability of ADHD in the high-IQ population: Results from the MGH longitudinal family studies of ADHD. *Journal of the American Academy of Child and Adolescent Psychiatry, 47*, 817-825.
24. Grossman, H., & Grossman, S. (1994). *Gender issues in education.* Boston: Allyn & Bacon.
25. O'Brien, J., Dowell, L., Mostofsky, S., Denckla, M., & Mahone, M. (2010). Neuropsychological profile of executive function in girls with attention-deficit/hyperactivity disorder. *Archives of Clinical Neuropsychology, 25*, 656-670.
26. Barkley, R. (2010). Deficient emotional self-regulation: A core component of attention-deficit/hyperactivity disorder. *Journal of ADHD and Related Disorders, 1*, 5-37.
27. Gilligan, C. (1982). *In a different voice: Psychological theory and women's development.* Cambridge, MA: Harvard University Press.
28. Crick, N. (1996). The role of overt aggression, relational aggression, and prosocial behaviour in the prediction of children's future social adjustment. *Child Development, 67,* 2-2.
29. Gaub, M., & Carlson, C. (1997). Gender differences in ADHD: A meta-analysis and critical review. *Journal of the American Academy of Child and Adolescent Psychiatry, 36*, 1036-1045.
30. Ohan, J., & Johnston, C. (2007). What is the social impact of ADHD in girls? A multi-method assessment. *Journal of Abnormal Child Psychology, 35*, 239-250.
31. Zalecki, C., & Hinshaw, S. (2004). Overt and relational aggression in girls with ADHD. *Journal of Clinical Child and Adolescent Psychology, 33*, 125-137.
32. Blachman, D., & Hinshaw, S. (2002). Patterns of friendship among girls with and without attention-deficit/hyperactivity disorder. *Journal of Abnormal Child Psychology, 30*, 625-640.
33. Zalecki, C., & Hinshaw, S. (2004). Overt and relational aggression in girls with ADHD. *Journal of Clinical Child and Adolescent Psychology, 33*, 125-137.
34. Zalecki, C., & Hinshaw, S. (2004). Overt and relational aggression in girls with ADHD. *Journal of Clinical Child and Adolescent Psychology, 33*, 125-137.
35. Ohan, J., & Johnston, C. (2007). What is the social impact of ADHD in girls? A multi-method assessment. *Journal of Abnormal Child Psychology, 35,* 239-250.

36. Ohan, J., & Johnston, C. (2011). Positive illusions of social competence in girls with and without ADHD. *Journal of Abnormal Child Psychology, 39*, 527-539.
37. Eisenberg, D., & Schneider, H. (2007). Perceptions of academic skills of children diagnosed with ADHD. *Journal of Attention Disorders, 10*, 390-397.
38. Blachman, D., & Hinshaw, S. (2002). Patterns of friendship among girls with and without attention-deficit/hyperactivity disorder. *Journal of Abnormal Child Psychology, 30*, 625-640.
39. Biederman, J., Petty, C., Monuteaux, M., Fried, R., Byrne, D., Mirto, T., Faraone, S., et al. (2010) Adult psychiatric outcomes of girls with attention deficit hyperactivity disorder: 11-year follow-up in a longitudinal case-control study. *American Journal of Psychiatry, 167*, 409-417.
40. Hinshaw, S., Owens, E., Zalecki, C., Huggins, S., Montenegro-Nevado, A., Schrodek, E., & Swanson, E. (2012). Prospective follow-up of girls with attention-deficit/hyperactivity disorder into early adulthood: Continuing impairment includes elevated risk for suicide attempts and self-injury. *Journal of Consulting and Clinical Psychology, 80*, 1041-1051.
41. Tannock, R. (1998). Attention deficit hyperactivity disorder: Advances in cognitive, neurobiological, and genetic research. *Journal of Child Psychology and Psychiatry, 39*, 65-99.
42. Woodward, L., Taylor, E., & Dowdney, L. (1998). The parenting and family functioning of children with hyperactivity. *Journal of Child Psychology and Psychiatry, 39*, 161-169.
43. Hinshaw, S. (2002). Preadolescent girls with attention-deficit/hyperactivity disorder: I. Background characteristics, comorbidity, cognitive and social functioning , and parenting practices. *Journal of Consulting and Clinical Psychology, 70*, 1086-1098.
44. Theule, J., Wiener, J., Tannock, R., & Jenkins, J. (2013). Parenting stress in families of children with ADHD: A meta-analysis. *Journal of Emotional and Behavioral Disorders, 21*, 3-17.
45. Peris, T., & Hinshaw, S. (2003). Family dynamics and preadolescent girls with ADHD: The relationship between expressed emotion, ADHD symptomatology, and comorbid disruptive behavior. *Journal of Child Psychology and Psychiatry, 44*, 1177-1190.
46. Hartung, C., Willcutt, E., Lahey, B., Pelham, W., Loney, J., Stein, M., & Keenan, K. (2002). Sex differences in young children who meet criteria for attention deficit hyperactivity disorder. *Journal of Clinical Adolescents Psychology, 4*, 453-464.
47. Staller, J., & Faraone, S. (2006). Attention deficit hyperactivity disorders in girls: Epidemiology and management. *CNS Drugs, 20*, 170-173.
48. Monuteaux, M., Fitzmaurice, G., Blacker, D., & Biederman, J. (2004) Specificity in the familial aggregation of overt and covert conduct disorder symptoms in a referred attention-deficit hyperactivity disorder sample. *Psychological Medicine, 34*, 1113-1127.
49. Faraone, S., Biederman, J., Spencer, T., Wilens, T., Seidman, L., Mick, E., & Doyle, A. (2000). Attention-deficit/hyperactivity disorder in adults: An overview. *Biological Psychiatry, 48*, 9-20.
50. Briscoe-Smith, A., & Hinshaw, S. (2006). Linkages between child abuse and attention-deficit/hyperactivity disorder in girls: Behavioral and social correlates. *Child Abuse and Neglect, 30*, 1239-1255.

CHAPTER FIVE

1. Hinshaw, S. P., Owens, E. B., Sami, N., & Fargeon, S. (2006). Prospective follow-up of girls with attention-deficit/hyperactivity disorder into adolescence: Evidence for continuing cross-domain impairment. *Journal of Consulting and Clinical Psychology, 74*, 489-499.
2. Barkley, R. (1998). *Attention deficit hyperactivity disorder: A handbook for diagnosis and treatment.* New York, NY: Guilford Press.

3. Hinshaw, S. P., Owens, E. B., Sami, N., & Fargeon, S. (2006). Prospective follow-up of girls with attention-deficit/hyperactivity disorder into adolescence: Evidence for continuing cross-domain impairment. *Journal of Consulting and Clinical Psychology, 74*, 489-499.
4. Abikoff, H., Jensen, P., Arnold, E., et al. (2002). Observed classroom behavior of children with ADHD: Relationship to gender and comorbidity. *Journal of Abnormal Child Psychology, 30*, 349-359.
5. Solden, S. (1995). *Women with attention deficit disorder*. Grass Valley, CA: Underwood Books.
6. Huessy, H. (1990). The pharmacotherapy of personality disorders in women. Paper presented at the Annual Meeting of the American Psychiatric Association (symposia), New York.
7. Elkins, I., Malone, S., Keyes, M., Iacono, W., & McGue, M. (2011). The impact of attention-deficit/hyperactivity disorder on preadolescent adjustment may be greater for girls than for boys. *Journal of Clinical and Child Adolescent Psychology, 40*, 532-545.
8. Miller, M., Ho, J., & Hinshaw, S. (2012). Executive functions in girls with ADHD followed prospectively into young adulthood. *Neuropsychology, 26*, 278-287.
9. Hinshaw, S., Owens, E., Zalecki, C., Huggins, S.P., Montenegro-Nevado, A., Schrodek, E., & Swanson, E. (2012). Prospective follow-up of girls with attention-deficit/hyperactivity disorder into early adulthood: Continuing impairment includes elevated risk for suicide attempts and self-injury. *Journal of Consulting and Clinical Psychology, 80*, 1041-1051.
10. Erikson, E. (1963). *Childhood and society* (Rev. ed.) New York: Norton.
11. American Association of University Women. (1991). *Shortchanging girls, shortchanging America: A call to action*. AAUW, Washington, DC.
12. Maccoby, E. (1998). *The two sexes: Growing up apart, coming together.* Harvard University Press.
13. Brown, L.M., & Gilligan, C. (1992). *Meeting at the crossroads: Women's psychology and girls' development*. Ballantine Books: New York.
14. Winnicott, D.W. (1964). *The child, the family, and the outside world*. London: Pelican Books.
15. Hoza, B. (2007). Peer functioning in children with ADHD. *Ambulatory Pediatrics, 7*, 101-106.
16. Wiener, J., & Mak, M. (2009). Peer victimization in children with attention-deficit/hyperactivity disorder. *Psychology in the Schools, 46*, 116-131.
17. Diamantopoulou, S., Rydell, A., Thorell, L. B., & Bohlin, G. (2007). Impact of executive functioning and symptoms of attention deficit hyperactivity disorder on children's peer relations and school performance. *Developmental Neuropsychology, 32*, 521–542.
18. Owens, E., Hinshaw, S., Lee, S., & Lahey, B. (2009). Few girls with childhood attention-deficit/hyperactivity disorder show positive adjustment during adolescence. *Journal of Clinical Child and Adolescent Psychology, 38*, 1–12.
19. Skogli, E., Teicher, M., Andersen, P., Hovik, K., & Oie, M. (2013). ADHD in girls and boys – gender differences in coexisting symptoms and executive function measures. *BMC Psychiatry, 13*, 298.
20. Biederman, J., Faraone, S.V., Spencer, T., Wilens, T., Mick, E., & Lapey, K.A. (1994). Gender differences in a sample of adults with attention deficit hyperactivity disorder. *Psychiatry Research, 53*, 13-29.
21. Hinshaw, S. (2002). Preadolescent girls with attention-deficit/hyperactivity disorder: I. Background characteristics, comorbidity, cognitive and social functioning, and parenting practices. *Journal of Consulting and Clinical Psychology, 70*, 1086-1098.
22. Staller, J., & Faraone, S. (2006). Attention deficit hyperactivity disorders in girls: Epidemiology and management. *CNS Drugs, 20*, 170-173.

23. Biederman, J., Monuteaux, M. C., Mick, E., Spencer, T., Wilens, T. E., Silva, J. M., Snyder, L., & Faraone, S. V. (2006). Young adult outcome of attention deficit hyperactivity disorder: A controlled 10-year follow-up study. *Psychological Medicine, 36*, 167-180.
24. Bauermeister, J. J., Shrout, P. E., Ramírez, R., Bravo, M., Alegría, M., Martínez-Taboas, A., Chavez, L., Rubio-Stipec, M., Garcia, P., Ribera, J., & Canino, G. (2007). ADHD correlates, comorbidity, and impairment in community and treated samples of children and adolescents. *Journal of Abnormal Child Psychology, 35*, 883-898.
25. Skogli, E., Teicher, M., Andersen, P., Hovik, K., & Oie, M. (2013). ADHD in girls and boys – gender differences in coexisting symptoms and executive function measures. *BMC Psychiatry, 13*, 298.
26. Bauermeister, J. J., Shrout, P. E., Ramírez, R., Bravo, M., Alegría, M., Martínez-Taboas, A., Chavez, L., Rubio-Stipec, M., Garcia, P., Ribera, J., & Canino, G. (2007). ADHD correlates, comorbidity, and impairment in community and treated samples of children and adolescents. *Journal of Abnormal Child Psychology, 35*, 883-898.
27. Biederman, J., Mick, E., & Faraone, S. (1998). Depression in attention deficit hyperactivity disorder (ADHD) in children: "True" depression or demoralization? *Journal of Affective Disorders, 47*, 113-122.
28. Hinshaw, S., Owens, E., Zalecki, C., Huggins, S.P., Montenegro-Nevado, A., Schrodek, E., & Swanson, E. (2012). Prospective follow-up of girls with attention-deficit/hyperactivity disorder into early adulthood: Continuing impairment includes elevated risk for suicide attempts and self-injury. *Journal of Consulting and Clinical Psychology, 80*, 1041-1051.
29. Becker, S., & Langberg, J. (2013). Sluggish cognitive tempo among young adolescents with ADHD relations to mental health, academic, and social functioning. *Journal of Attention Disorders, 17*, 681-689.
30. Skogli, E., Teicher, M., Andersen, P., Hovik, K., & Oie, M. (2013). ADHD in girls and boys – gender differences in coexisting symptoms and executive function measures. *BMC Psychiatry, 13*, 298.
31. Skogli, E., Teicher, M., Andersen, P., Hovik, K., & Oie, M. (2013). ADHD in girls and boys – gender differences in coexisting symptoms and executive function measures. *BMC Psychiatry, 13*, 298.
32. Monuteaux, M. C., Fitzmaurice, G., Blacker, D., Buka, S. L., & Biederman, J. (2004). Specificity in the familial aggregation of overt and covert conduct disorder symptoms in a referred attention-deficit hyperactivity disorder sample. *Psychological Medicine, 34*, 1113-1127.
33. Hartung, C., Willcutt, E., Lahey, B., Pelham, W., Loney, J., Stein, M., & Keenan, K. (2002). Sex differences in young children who meet criteria for attention deficit hyperactivity disorder. *Journal of Clinical Adolescent Psychology, 4*, 453-464.
34. Staller, J., & Faraone, S. (2006). Attention deficit hyperactivity disorders in girls: Epidemiology and management. *CNS Drugs, 20*, 170-173.
35. Huessy, H. (1990). The pharmacotherapy of personality disorders in women. Paper presented at the Annual Meeting of the American Psychiatric Association (symposia), New York.
36. Jacobson, L., Williford, A., & Planta, R. (2011). The role of executive function in children's competent adjustment to middle school. *Child Neuropsychology, 17*, 255-280.
37. Hinshaw, S. (2002). Preadolescent girls with attention-deficit/hyperactivity disorder: I. Background characteristics, comorbidity, cognitive and social functioning, and parenting practices. *Journal of Consulting and Clinical Psychology, 70*, 1086-1098.
38. Hinshaw, S., Carte, E., Fan, C., Jassy, J., & Owens, E. (2007). Neuropsychological functioning of girls with attention-deficit/hyperactivity disorder followed prospectively into adolescence: Evidence for continuing deficits? *Neuropsychology, 21*, 263-273.

39. Pingault, J., Tremblay, R., Vitaro, F., Carbonneau, R., Genolini, C., Falissard, B., & Côté, S. (2011). Childhood trajectories of inattention and hyperactivity and prediction of educational attainment in early adulthood: A 16-year longitudinal population-based study. *American Journal of Psychiatry, 168*, 1164-1170.
40. Biederman, J., Monuteaux, M., Doyle, A., Seidman, L. J., Wilens, T. E., Ferrero, F., Morgan, C., & Faraone, S. V. (2004). Impact of executive function deficits and attention-deficit/hyperactivity disorder (ADHD) on academic outcomes in children. *Journal of Consulting and Clinical Psychology, 72*, 757-766.
41. Biederman, J., Petty, C. R., Monuteaux, M. C., Mick, E., Parcell, T., Westerberg, D., & Faraone, S. V. (2008). The longitudinal course of comorbid oppositional defiant disorder in girls with ADHD: Findings from a controlled 5-year prospective longitudinal follow-up study. *Journal of Developmental and Behavioral Pediatrics, 29*, 501-507 .
42. Elkins, I., Malone, S., Keyes, M., Iacono, W., & McGue, M. (2011). The impact of attention-deficit/hyperactivity disorder on preadolescent adjustment may be greater for girls than for boys. *Journal of Clinical and Child Adolescent Psychology, 40*, 532-545
43. Seidman, L., Biederman, J., Monuteaux, M., et al. (2005). Impact of gender and age on executive functioning: Do girls and boys with and without attention deficit hyperactivity disorder differ neuropsychologically in preteen and teenage years? *Developmental Neuropsychology, 27*, 79-105.
44. Gershon, J. (2002). Gender differences in ADHD. *The ADHD Report, 10*, 8-16.
45. Yoshimatsu, K., Barbaresi, W., Colligan, R., Killian, J., Voigt, R., Weaver, A., & Katusic, S. (2011). Written-language disorder among children with and without ADHD in a population-based birth cohort. *Pediatrics, 128*, e605-e612.
46. O'Brien, J., Dowell, L., Mostofsky, S., Denckla, M., & Mahone, E. (2010). Neuropsychological profile of executive function in girls with attention-deficit/hyperactivity disorder. *Archives of Clinical Neuropsychology, 25*, 656-670.
47. Wodka, E., Mostofsky, S., Prahme, C., Gidley Larson, J. C., Loftis, C., Denckla, M. B., & Mark Mahone, E. (2008). Process examination of executive function in ADHD: Sex and subtype effects. *The Clinical Neuropsychologist, 22*, 826-841.
48. Hinshaw, S. (2002). Preadolescent girls with attention-deficit/hyperactivity disorder: I. Background characteristics, comorbidity, cognitive and social functioning, and parenting practices. *Journal of Consulting and Clinical Psychology, 70*, 1086-1098.
49. Coles, E., Slavec, J., Bernstein, M., & Baroni, E. (2012). Exploring the gender gap in referrals for children with ADHD and other disruptive behavior disorders. *Journal of Attention Disorders, 16*, 101-108.
50. Quinn, P., & Wigal, S. (2004). Perceptions of girls and ADHD: Results from a national survey. *Medscape General Medicine, 6*, 2.
51. Skogli, E., Teicher, M., Andersen, P., Hovik, K., & Oie, M. (2013). ADHD in girls and boys – gender differences in coexisting symptoms and executive function measures. *BMC Psychiatry, 13*, 298.
52. Biederman, J., Faraone, S., Mick, E., Williamson, S., Wilens, T., Spencer, T., Weber, W., Jetton, J., Kraus, I., Pert, J., & Zallen, B. (1999). Clinical correlates of ADHD in females: Findings from a large group of girls ascertained from pediatric and psychiatric referral sources. *Journal of the American Academy of Child and Adolescent Psychiatry, 38*, 966-975.
53. Brown, T., Reichel, P., & Quinlan, D. (2011). Executive function impairments in high IQ children and adolescents with ADHD. *Open Journal of Psychiatry*, 1, 56-65.
54. Antshel, K., Faraone, S., et al. (2007). Is attention deficit hyperactivity disorder a valid diagnosis in the presence of high IQ? Results from the MGH longitudinal family studies of ADHD. *Journal of Child Psychology and Psychiatry, 48*, 687-694.
55. Brown, T., Reichel, P., & Quinlan, D. (2011). Executive function impairments in high IQ children and adolescents with ADHD. *Open Journal of Psychiatry, 1*, 56-65

56. Rinsky, J., & Hinshaw, S. (2011). Linkages between childhood executive functioning and adolescent social functioning and psychopathology in girls with ADHD. *Child Neuropsychology, 17*, 368-390.
57. Wiener, J., & Mak, M. (2009). Peer victimization in children with Attention-Deficit/Hyperactivity Disorder. *Psychology in the Schools, 46*, 116-131.
58. Sciberras, E., Ohan, J., & Anderson, V. (2012). Bullying and peer victimization in adolescent girls with attention-deficit/hyperactivity disorder. *Child Psychiatry and Human Development, 43*, 254-270.
59. Hinshaw, S. (2002). Preadolescent girls with attention-deficit/hyperactivity disorder: I. Background characteristics, comorbidity, cognitive and social functioning, and parenting practices. *Journal of Consulting and Clinical Psychology, 70*, 1086-1098
60. Abikoff, H., Jensen, P., Arnold, E., et al. (2002). Observed classroom behavior of children with ADHD: Relationship to gender and comorbidity. *Journal of Abnormal Child Psychology, 30*, 349-359.
61. Rucklidge, J.J. (2010). Gender differences in attention-deficit/hyperactivity disorder. *Psychiatric Clinic of North America, 33*, 357-373.
62. Abikoff, H., Jensen, P., Arnold, E., et al. (2002). Observed classroom behavior of children with ADHD: Relationship to gender and comorbidity. *Journal of Abnormal Child Psychology, 30*, 349-359.
63. Zalecki, C., & Hinshaw, S. (2004). Overt and relational aggression in girls with attention deficit hyperactivity disorder. *Journal of Clinical Child and Adolescent Psychiatry, 33*, 125-137.
64. Crick, N. R., Ostrov, J. M., & Werner, N. E. (2006). A longitudinal study of relational aggression, physical aggression, and children's social–psychological adjustment. *Journal of Abnormal Child Psychology, 34,* 127-138.
65. Elkins, I., Malone, S., Keyes, M., Iacono, W., & McGue, M. (2011). The impact of attention-deficit/hyperactivity disorder on preadolescent adjustment may be greater for girls than for boys. *Journal of Clinical and Child Adolescent Psychology, 40*, 532-545.
66. McQuade, J. D., & Hoza, B. (2008). Peer problems in attention deficit hyperactivity disorder: Current status and future directions. *Developmental Disabilities Research Reviews, 14*, -.
67. Rose, A., & Rudolph, K. (2006). A review of sex differences in peer relationship processes: Potential trade-offs for the emotional and development of girls and boys. *Psychological Bulletin, 132*, 98–131.
68. Ohan, J., & Johnston, C. (2007). What is the social impact of ADHD in girls? A multi-method assessment. *Journal of Abnormal Child Psychology, 35*, 239-250.
69. Grotpeter, J., & Crick, N. (1996). Relational aggression, overt aggression, and friendship. *Child Development, 67,* 2-2.
70. Cardoos, S., & Hinshaw, S. (2011). Friendship as protection from peer victimization for girls with and without ADHD. *Journal of Abnormal Child Psychology, 39*, 1035-1045.
71. Becker, S., Fite, P., Luebbe, A., Stoppelbein, L., & Greening, L. (2013). Friendship intimacy exchange buffers the relation between ADHD symptoms and later social problems among children attending an after-school care program. *Journal of Psychopathological Behavioral Assessment, 35*, 142-152.
72. Mrug, S., Molina, B., Hoza, B., Gerdes, A., Hinshaw, S., Hechtman, L., & Arnold, L. (2012). Peer rejection and friendships in children with attention-deficit/hyperactivity disorder: Contributions to long-term outcomes. *Journal of Abnormal Child Psychology, 40*, 1013-1026.
73. Crick, N. R. (1997). Engagement in gender normative versus nonnormative forms of aggression: Links to social–psychological adjustment. *Developmental Psychology, 33*, 610-617.

74. Mikami, A. Y., & Hinshaw, S. P. (2006). Resilient adolescent adjustment among girls: Buffers of childhood peer rejection and attention-deficit/hyperactivity disorder. *Journal of Abnormal Child Psychology, 34*, 823-837.
75. Levine, M., Smolak, L., & Hayden, H. (1994). The relation of sociocultural factors to eating attitudes and behaviors among middle school girls. *The Journal of Early Adolescence, 14*, 471-490.
76. Pipher, M. (1994). *Reviving Ophelia.* Ballantine Publishing Group
77. Salmivalli, C., Sainio, M., & Hodges, E. (2013). Electronic victimization: Correlates, antecedents, and consequences among elementary and middle school students. *Journal of Clinical Child and Adolescent Psychology, 42*, 442-453.
78. Weiss, M., Baer, S., Allan, B., Saran, K., & Schibuk, H. (2011). The screens culture: Impact on ADHD. *Attention Deficit and Hyperactivity Disorders, 3*, -.
79. Huessy, H. (1990). The pharmacotherapy of personality disorders in women. Paper presented at the Annual Meeting of the American Psychiatric Association (symposia), New York.

CHAPTER SIX

1. Fischer, M., Barkley, R.A., Fletcher, K.E., & Smallish, L. (1993). The adolescent outcome of hyperactive children: Predictors of psychiatric, academic, social, and emotional adjustment. *Journal of the American Academy of Child and Adolescent Psychiatry, 32*, -.
2. Biederman, J., Monuteaux, M.C., Mick, E., Spencer, T., Wilens, T.E., Silva, J.M., Snyder, L.E., & Faraone, S.V. (2006). Young adult outcome of attention deficit hyperactivity disorder: A controlled 10-year follow-up study. *Psychological Medicine, 36*, 167-179.
3. Biederman, J., Petty, C.R., Evans, M., Small, J., & Faraone, S.V. (2010). How persistent is ADHD? A controlled 10-year follow-up study of boys with ADHD. *Psychiatry Research, 177*, 299-304.
4. Biederman, J., Petty, C.R., Monuteaux, M.C., Fried, R., Byrne, D., Mirto, T., Spencer, T., Wilens, T.E., & Faraone, S.V. (2010). Adult psychiatric outcomes of girls with attention deficit hyperactivity disorder: 11-year follow-up in a longitudinal case-control study. *American Journal of Psychiatry, 167*, 409-417.
5. Hinshaw, S.P., Owens, E.B., Sami, N., & Fargeon, S. (2006). Prospective follow-up of girls with attention-deficit/hyperactivity disorder into adolescence: Evidence for continuing cross-domain impairment. *Journal of Consulting and Clinical Psychology, 74(3)*, 489-499.
6. Wolraich, M.L., Wibbelsman, C.J., Brown, T.E., Evans, S.W., Gotlieb, E.M., Knight, J.R., Ross, E.C., Shubiner, H.H., Wender, E.H., & Wilens, T. (2005). Attention-deficit/hyperactivity disorder among adolescents: A review of the diagnosis, treatment, and clinical implications. *Pediatrics, 115*, 1734-1746.
7. Lee, S.S., Lahey, B.B., Owens, E.B., & Hinshaw, S.P. (2008). Few preschool boys and girls with ADHD are well-adjusted during adolescence. *Journal of Abnormal Child Psychology, 36*, 373-383.
8. Owens, E.B., Hinshaw, S.P., Lee, L.L., & Lahey, B.B. (2009). Few girls with children ADHD show positive adjustment during adolescence. *Journal of Clinical Child and Adolescent Psychology, 38*, 132-143.
9. Owens, E.B., Hinshaw, S.P., Lee, L.L., & Lahey, B.B. (2009). Few girls with children ADHD show positive adjustment during adolescence. *Journal of Clinical Child and Adolescent Psychology, 38*, 132-143.
10. Sibley, M.H., Altszuler, A.R., Morrow, A.S., & Merrill, B.M. (2014). Mapping the academic problem behaviors of adolescents with ADHD *School Psychology Quarterly, Jun 16.*
11. Hinshaw, S.P., Carte, E. T., Fan, C., Jassy, J.S., & Owens, E.B. (2007). Neuropsychological functioning of girls with attention-deficit/hyperactivity disorder followed prospectively into adolescence: Evidence for continuing deficits? *Neuropsychology, 21*, 263-273.

12. Miller, M., Ho, J., & Hinshaw, S.P. (2012). Executive functions in girls with ADHD followed prospectively into young adulthood. *Neuropsychology, 26,* 278-287.
13. Babinski, D.E., Sibley, M.H., Ross, J.M., & Pelham, W.E. (2013). The effects of single versus mixed gender treatment for adolescent girls with ADHD. *Journal of Clinical Child and Adolescent Psychology, 42,* 243-250.
14. Hinshaw, S., & Krantz, R. (2009). *The triple bind: Saving our teenage girls from today's pressures and conflicting expectations.* New York: Ballantine Books.
15. Abikoff, H.B., Jensen, P.S., Arnold, L.L., Hoza, B., et al. (2002). Observed classroom behavior of children with ADHD: Relationship to gender and comorbidity. *Journal of Abnormal Child Psychology, 30,* 349-359.
16. Huessy, H.R. (1990). The pharmacotherapy of personality disorders in women. Paper presented at the annual meeting of the American Psychiatric Association (symposia), New York.
17. American Psychiatric Association. (2013). *Diagnostic and statistical manual of mental disorders, Fifth edition.* Washington, DC.
18. Ohan, J., & Visser, T. (2009). Why is there a gender gap in children presenting for attention deficit/hyperactivity disorder services? *Journal of Clinical Child and Adolescent Psychology, 38,* 650-660.
19. Biederman, J., Ball, S.W., Monuteaux, M.C., Mick, E., Spencer, T.J., et al. (2008). New insights into the comorbidity between ADHD and major depression in adolescent and young adult females. *Journal of the American Academy of Child and Adolescent Psychiatry, 47,* 426-434.
20. Biederman, J., Petty, C.R., Monuteaux, M.C., Fried, R., Byrne, D., Mirto, T., Spencer, T., Wilens, T.E., & Faraone, S.V. (2010). Adult psychiatric outcomes of girls with attention deficit hyperactivity disorder: 11-year follow-up in a longitudinal case-control study. *American Journal of Psychiatry, 167,* 409-417.
21. Hinshaw, S.P., Owens, E.B., Sami, N., & Fargeon, S. (2006). Prospective follow-up of girls with attention-deficit/hyperactivity disorder into adolescence: Evidence for continuing cross-domain impairment. *Journal of Consulting and Clinical Psychology, 74(3),* 489-499.
22. Hinshaw, S.P., Owens, E.B., Zalecki, C., Huggins, S.P. et al. (2012). Prospective follow-up of girls with attention-deficit/hyperactivity disorder into early adulthood: Continuing impairment includes elevated risk for suicide attempts and self-injury. *Journal Consulting and Clinical Psychology, 80,* 1041-1051.
23. Quinn, P., & Wigal, S. (2004). Perceptions of girls and ADHD: Results from a national survey. *Medscape General Medicine, 6,* 2.
24. Hinshaw, S., & Krantz, R. (2009). *The triple bind: Saving our teenage girls from today's pressures and conflicting expectations.* New York: Ballantine Books.
25. Pliszka, S.R. (1998). Comorbidity of attention-deficit/hyperactivity disorder with psychiatric disorder: An overview. *Journal of Clinical Psychiatry, 59, Suppl 7,* 50-58.
26. Monuteaux, M.C., Faraone, S.V., Michelle Gross, L., & Biederman, J. (2007). Predictors, clinical characteristics, and outcome of conduct disorder in girls with attention-deficit/hyperactivity disorder: A longitudinal study. *Psychological Medicine, 37,* 1731-1741.
27. Arnold, L.E. (1996). Sex differences in ADHD: Conference summary. *Journal of Abnormal Child Psychology, 24,* 555-569.
28. Barkley, R.A., Fischer, M., Smallish, L., & Fletcher, K. (2006). Young adult outcome of hyperactive children: Adaptive functioning in major life activities. *Journal of the American Academy of Child and Adolescent Psychiatry, 45,* 192-202.
29. Quinn, P., & Wigal, S. (2004). Perceptions of girls and ADHD: Results from a national survey. *Medscape General Medicine, 6,* 2.
30. Huggins, S.P., Rooney, M.E., & Chronis-Tuscano, A. (2012). Risky sexual behavior among college students with ADHD: Is the mother-child relationship protective? *Journal of Attention Disorders,* 1087054712459560, first published on October 9, 2012.

31. Hosain, G.M., Berenson, A.B., Tennen, H., Bauer, L.O., & Wu, Z.H. (2012). Attention deficit hyperactivity symptoms and risky sexual behavior in young adult women. *Journal of Womens' Health, 21(4)*, 463-468.
32. Lehti, V., Niemela, S., Heinze, M., Sillanmaki, L., Helenius, H., Piha, J., Kumpulainen, K., Tamminen, T., Almqvist, F., & Sourander, A. (2012), Childhood predictors of becoming a teenage mother among Finnish girls. *Acta Obstet Gynecol Scand, 91*,1-1.
33. Beck, N., Warnke, A., Kruger, H.P., & Barglik, W. (1996). Hyperkinetic syndrome and behavioral disorders in street traffic: A case controlled pilot study. Klinik und Poliklinik fur Kinder-und Jugendpsychiatrie, Julius Maximilians Z. *Kinder Jugerpsychiatrie, 24(2)*, 82-91.
34. Nada-Raja, S., Langley, J.D., McGee, R., Williams, S.M., et al. (1997). Inattentive and hyperactive behaviors and driving offenses in adolescence: Health Research Council of New Zealand. *Journal of the American Academy of Child and Adolescent Psychiatry, 36*, 512-522.
35. Biederman, J., Ball, S.W., Monuteaux, M.C., Mick, E., Spencer, T.J., et al. (2008). New insights into the comorbidity between ADHD and major depression in adolescent and young adult females. *Journal of the American Academy of Child and Adolescent Psychiatry, 47*, 426-434.
36. Biederman, J., Ball, S.W., Monuteaux, M.C., Mick, E., Spencer, T.J., et al. (2008). New insights into the comorbidity between ADHD and major depression in adolescent and young adult females. *Journal of the American Academy of Child and Adolescent Psychiatry, 47*, 426-434.
37. Chronis-Tuscano, A., Molina, B.S.G., Pelham, W.E., Applegate, B., Dahlke, A., Overmeyer, M., & Lahey, B. (2010). Very early predictors of adolescent depression and suicide attempts in children with attention-deficit/hyperactivity disorder. *Archives of General Psychiatry, 67*, 1044–1051.
38. Seymour, K.E., Chronis-Tuscano, A., Halldorsdottir, T., Stupica, B., Owens, K., & Sacks, T. (2012). Emotion regulation mediates the relationship between ADHD and depressive symptoms in youth. *Journal of Abnormal Child Psychology, 40*, 595–606.
39. Hinshaw, S.P., Owens, E.B., Zalecki, C., Huggins, S.P. et al. (2012). Prospective follow-up of girls with attention-deficit/hyperactivity disorder into early adulthood: Continuing impairment includes elevated risk for suicide attempts and self-injury. *Journal Consulting and Clinical Psychology, 80*, 1041-1051.
40. Swanson, E.N., Owens, E.B., & Hinshaw, S.P. (2014). Pathways to self-harmful behaviors in young women with and without ADHD: A longitudinal examination of mediating factors. *Journal of Child Psychology and Psychiatry, 55*, 505–515.
41. Biederman, J., Ball, S.W., & Monuteaux, M.C. (2007). Are girls with ADHD at risk for eating disorders? Results from a controlled, five-year prospective study. *Journal of Developmental and Behavioral Pediatrics, 28*, 302–307
42. Mikami, A.Y., Hinshaw, S.P., Patterson, K.A., & Lee, J.C. (2008). Eating pathology among adolescent girls with attention-deficit/hyperactivity disorder. *Journal of Abnormal Psychology, 117*, 225–235.
43. Dukarm, C. (2005). Bulimia nervosa and ADD: A possible role for stimulant medication. *Journal of Women's Health, 14,* 345–350.
44. Sibley, M.H., Pelham, W.E., Molina, B.S., Coxe, S., Kipp, H., Gnagy, E.M., Meinzer, M., Ross, J.M., & Lahey, B.B. (2014). The role of early childhood ADHD and subsequent CD in the initiation and escalation of adolescent cigarette, alcohol, and marijuana use. *Journal of Abnormal Psychology, 123,* 362-374.
45. Ostojic, D., Charach, A., Henderson, J., McAuley, T., & Crosbie, J. (2014). Childhood ADHD and addictive behaviours in adolescence: A canadian sample. *Journal of the Canadian Academy of Child and Adolescent Psychiatry, 23*, 128-135.
46. Biederman, J., Faraone, S.V., Mick, E., Williamson, S., Wilens, T.E., Spencer, T.J., Weber, W., Jetton, J., Kraus, I., Pert, J., & Zallen, B. (1999). Clinical correlates of ADHD in females: Findings from a large group of girls ascertained from pediatric and psychiatric referral

sources. *Journal of the American Academy of Child and Adolescent Psychiatry, 38*, 966-975. 47. Solden, S. (1995). *Women with attention deficit disorder.* Grass Valley CA: Underwood Books.

CHAPTER SEVEN

1. Kopp, S., Beckung, E., & Gillberg, C. (2010). Developmental coordination disorder and other motor control problems in girls with autism spectrum disorder and/or attention-deficit/hyperactivity disorder. *Research in Developmental Disabilities, 31*, 350-361.
2. Fliers, E., Rommelse, N., Vermeulen, S.H., et al. (2008). Motor coordination problems in children and adolescents with ADHD rated by parents and teachers: Effects of age and gender. *Journal of Neural Transmission, 115*, 211-220.
3. Riccio, C.A., Hynd, G.W., Cohen, M.J., Hall, J., & Molt, L. (1994). Comorbidity of central auditory processing disorder and attention-deficit hyperactivity disorder. *Journal of the American Academy of Child and Adolescent Psychiatry, 33*, 849-857.
4. Riccio, C.A., Hynd, G.W., Cohen, M.J., Hall, J., & Molt, L. (1994). Comorbidity of central auditory processing disorder and attention-deficit hyperactivity disorder. *Journal of the American Academy of Child and Adolescent Psychiatry, 33*, 849-857.
5. Helland, W., Biringer, E., Helland, T., & Heimann, M. (2012). Exploring language profiles for children with ADHD and children with asperger syndrome. *Journal of Attention Disorders, 16*, 34-43.
6. Spencer, T., Biederman, J., Harding, M., et al. (1998). Disentangling the overlap between Tourette's disorder and ADHD. *Journal of Child Psychology and Psychiatry, 39*, 1037-1044.
7. Freeman, R.D. (2007). Tic disorders and ADHD: Answers from a world-wide clinical dataset on Tourette syndrome. *European Child and Adolescent Psychiatry, 16*, 15-23.
8. Gillberg, C., Gillberg, I.C., Rasmussen, P., Kadesjo, B., Soderstrom, H., Rastam, M., Johnson, M., Rothenberger, A., & Niklasson, L. (2004). Coexisting disorders in ADHD- implications for diagnosis and intervention. *European Child and Adolescent Psychiatry, 13*, 180–192.
9. American Psychiatric Association. (2013). *Diagnostic and statistical manual of mental disorders, Fifth edition.* Arlington, VA: American Psychiatric Publishers.
10. Gould, J., & Ashton-Smith, J. (2011). Missed diagnosis or misdiagnosis: Girls and women on the autism spectrum. *Good Autism Practice, 12*, 34-41.
11. Kopp, S., & Gilberg, C. (2011). The autism spectrum screening questionnaire (ASSQ)-revised extended version (ASSQ-REV): An instrument for better capturing the autism phenotype in girls? A preliminary study involving 191 clinical cases and community controls. *Research in Developmental Disabilities, 32*, 2875-2888.
12. Kotte, A., Joshi, G., Fried, R., et al. (2013). Autistic traits in children with and without ADHD. *Pediatrics, 132*, e612-622.
13. Caamano, M., Boada, L., Moreno, C., et al. (2013). Psychopathology in children and adolescents with ASD without mental retardation. *Journal of Autism and Developmental Disorders, 43*, 2442-2449.
14. Gillberg, C., Gillberg, I.C., Rasmussen, P., Kadesjo, B., Soderstrom, H., Rastam, M., Johnson, M., Rothenberger, A., & Niklasson, L. (2004). Coexisting disorders in ADHD—implications for diagnosis and intervention. *European Child and Adolescent Psychiatry, 13*, 180–192.
15. Sexton, C.C., Gelhorn, H.L., Bell, J.A., & Classi, P.M. (2012). The co-occurrence of reading disorder and ADHD: Epidemiology, treatment, psychosocial impact, and economic burden. *Journal of Learning Disabilities,45*, 538-564.
16. Sexton, C.C., Gelhorn, H.L., Bell, J.A., & Classi, P.M. (2012). The co-occurrence of reading disorder and ADHD: Epidemiology, treatment, psychosocial impact, and economic burden. *Journal of Learning Disabilities,45*, 538-564.

17. Yoshimasu, K., Barbaresi, W.J., Colligan, R.C., et al. (2011). Written-language disorder among children with and without ADHD in a population-based birth cohort. *Pediatrics, 128,* 3605-3612.
18. Miller, M., Loya, F., & Hinshaw, S. P. (2013). Executive functions in girls with and without childhood ADHD: Developmental trajectories and associations with symptom change. *Journal of Child Psychology & Psychiatry, 54,* 1005-1015.

CHAPTER EIGHT

1. Barkley, R. (2012). *Executive functions: What they are, how they work, and why they evolved.* New York: Guilford Press.
2. Blair, C., & Razza, R.P. (2007). Relating effortful control, executive function, and false belief understanding to emerging math and literacy ability in kindergarten. *Child Development, 78,* 647-663.
3. Ruff, H., & Rothbard, M.K. (1996). *Attention in early development: Themes and variations.* New York, NY: Oxford University Press.
4. Mischel, W., Ayduk, O., Berman, M.G., et al. (2011). 'Willpower' over the lifespan: Decomposing self-regulation. *Social Cognitive and Affective Neuroscience, 6,* 252-256.
5. Bodrova, E., & Leong, D.J. (2007). *Tools of the mind: The Vygotskian approach to early childhood education, edition 2.* New York: Merrill/Prentice Hall; 2007.
6. Vygotsky LS. (1978). *Mind in society: The development of higher psychological processes.* Cambridge: Harvard University Press.
7. Diamond, A. & Lee, K. (2011). Interventions shown to aid executive function development in children 4-12 years old. *Science,* , 959–964.
8. Hinshaw, S.P. (2002) Preadolescent girls with attention-deficit/hyperactivity disorder: 1. Background characteristics, comorbidity, cognitive and social functioning, and parenting practices. *Journal of Consulting and Clinical Psychology, 70,* 1086-1098.
9. Rinsky, J.R. & Hinshaw, S. (2011). Linkages between childhood executive functioning and adolescent social functioning and psychopathology in girls with ADHD. *Child Neuropsychology, 17,* 368-390.

CHAPTER NINE

1. Hartmann, T. (2003). *The Edison Gene: ADHD and the gift of the hunter child.* Rochester, VT: Inner Traditions/Bear & Company.
2. Hartmann, T. (2003). *The Edison Gene: ADHD and the gift of the hunter child.* Rochester, VT: Inner Traditions/Bear & Company.
3. Matthews, J., Ponitz, C., & Morrison, F. (2009). Early gender differences in self-regulation and academic achievement. *Journal of Educational Psychology, 101,* 689-704.
4. Abikoff, H., Jensen, P., Arnold, L.E., Hoza, B., Hechtman, L., Pollack, S., Martin, D., Alvir, J., March, J., Hinshaw, S., et al. (2002). Observed classroom behavior of children with ADHD: Relationship to gender and comorbidity. *Journal of Abnormal Child Psychology, 30,* 349-359.
5. Antshel, K.M., Faraone, S.V., Stallone, K., Nave, A., Kaufmann, F., Doyle, A., Fried, R., Seidman, L., & Biederman, J. (2007). Is attention deficit hyperactivity disorder a valid diagnosis in the presence of high IQ? Results from the MGH Longitudinal Family Studies of ADHD. *Journal of Child Psychology and Psychiatry, 48,* 687–694.
6. Stevenson, J., Langley, K., Pay, H., Payton, A., Worthington, J., Ollier, W., & Thapar, A. (2005). Attention deficit hyperactivity disorder with reading disabilities: Preliminary genetic findings on the involvement of the ADRA2A gene. *Journal of Child Psychology and Psychiatry, 46,* 1081-1088.

7. Willcutt, E.G., & Pennington, B.F. (2000). Comorbidity of reading disability and attention-deficit/hyperactivity disorder differences by gender and subtype. *Journal of Learning Disabilities, 33*, 179-191.
8. Yoshimasu, K., Barbaresi, W., Colligan, R., et al. (2011). Written-language disorder among children with and without ADHD in a population-based birth cohort. *Pediatrics, 128*, e605-612.
9. Cutting, L.E., Koth, C.W., Mahone, M., & Denckla, M.B. (2003). Evidence for unexpected weaknesses in learning in children with attention-deficit/hyperactivity disorder without reading disabilities. *Journal of Learning Disabilities, 36*, 259-269.
10. Miller, M., & Hinshaw, S. P. (2010). Does childhood executive function predict adolescent functional outcomes in girls with ADHD? *Journal of Abnormal Child Psychology, 38*, -.
11. Miller, M., Nevado-Montenegro, A. J., & Hinshaw, S. P. (2012). Childhood executive function continues to predict outcomes in young adult females with and without childhood-diagnosed ADHD. *Journal of Abnormal Child Psychology, 40*, 657-668.
12. Imeraj, L., Antrop, I., Sonuga-Barke, E., Deboutte, D., Deschepper, E., Bal, S., & Roeyers, H. (2013). The impact of instructional context on classroom on-task behavior: A matched comparison of children with ADHD and non-ADHD classmates. *Journal of School Psychology, 51*, 487-498.
13. Albrecht, N. (2012). Mindfully teaching in the classroom: A literature review. *Australian Journal of Teacher Education, 37*, 1-14.
14. Diamond, A., & Lee, K. (2011). Interventions shown to aid executive function development in children 4-12 years old. *Science*, , 959-964.
15. Bierman K.L., Coie, J.D., Dodge, K.A., Greenberg, M.T., Lockman, J.E., McMahon, R.J., & Pinderhughes, E. (2010). The effects of a multiyear universal social-emotional learning program: The role of student and school characteristics. *Journal of Consulting and Clinical Psychology, 78*, 156-168.
16. Chacko, A., Bedard, A.C., Marks, D.J., Feirsen, N., Uderman, J.Z., Chimiklis, A., Rajwan, E., Cornwell, M., Anderson, L., Zwilling, A., andRamon, M. (2013). A randomized clinical trial of Cogmed Working Memory Training in school-age children with ADHD: A replication in a diverse sample using a control condition. *The Journal of Child Psychology and Psychiatry, 55*, 247-253.
17. Kercood, S., Zentall, S. S., Vinh, M., & Tom-Wright, K. (2012). Attentional cuing in math word problems for girls at-risk for ADHD and their peers in general education settings. *Contemporary Educational Psychology, 37*, 106-112.
18. Barron, K. E., Evans, S. W., Baranik, L. E., Serpell, Z. N., & Buvinger, E. (2006). Achievement goals of students with ADHD. *Learning Disability Quarterly, 29*, 137–158.
19. Cacioppo, J., & Hawkley, L.D. (2009). Perceived social isolation and cognition. *Trends in Cognitive Science, 13*, 447-454.
20. Kramer, J. H., Knee, K., & Delis, D. C. (2000). Verbal memory impairments in dyslexia. *Archives of Clinical Neuropsychology, 15*, 83–93.
21. Cacioppo, J.T., Hawkley, L. C., Leary, M. R. (Ed). & Hoyle, R. H. (Ed). (2009). *Handbook of individual differences in social behavior*, (pp 227-240). New Your, NY: Guilford Press, xv, 624 pp
22. Diamond, A., & Lee, K. (2008). Interventions shown to aid executive function development in children 4-12 years old. *Science*, , 959-964.
23. Ratey, J., & Hagerman, E. (2008). *Spark: The revolutionary new science of exercise and the brain*. Boston: Little, Brown & Company.
24. Duvall, S.F., Delquadri, J.C., & Ward, D.L. (2004). Preliminary investigation of the effectiveness of homeschool instructional environment for students with attention-deficit/hyperactivity disorder. *School Psychology Review, 33*, 140-158.

CHAPTER TEN

1. Kinsbourne, M. (1992). Quality of life in children with ADHD. *Challenge, 6*, 1-2.
2. Arcia, E., & Conners, C.K. (1998). Gender differences in ADHD? *Journal of Developmental and Behavioral Pediatrics, 19*, 77-83.
3. Hinshaw, S. P. (1994). *Attention deficits and hyperactivity in children.* Thousand Oaks, CA: Sage.
4. The MTA Cooperative Group. (1999). A 14-month randomized clinical trial of treatment strategies for attention-deficit/hyperactivity disorder. *Archives of General Psychiatry, 56*, 1073-1086.
5. A.D.H.D. Experts Re-evaluate Study's Zeal for Drugs Alan Schwartz, Dec. 29, 2013, Health Section, New York Times.
6. Nadeau, K. (1998). *Help4ADD@HighSchool.* Silver Spring, MD: Advantage Books.
7. Miano, S. (2013). Introduction to the special section on sleep and ADHD. *Journal of Attention Disorders, 17*, 547-549.
8. Owens, J., Gruber, R., Brown, T., et al. (2012). Future research directions in sleep and ADHD: Report of a consensus working group. *Journal of Attention Disorders, 17*, 550-564.
9. Ratey, J. (2013). *Spark: The revolutionary new science of exercise and the brain.* Little, Brown and Company.
10. Salmon, P. (2001). Effects of physical exercise on anxiety, depression, and sensitivity to stress: A unifying theory. *Clinical Psychiatric Review, 21*, 33-61.
11. Howard, A.L., Robinson, M., Smith, G. J., et al. (2012). ADHD is associated with a Western dietary pattern in adolescents. *Journal of Attention Disorders, 15*, 403-411.
12. Conners, C.K., & Blouin, A.G. (1983). Nutritional effects on behavior of children. *Journal of Psychiatric Research, 17*, 193–201.
13. Mahoney, C.R., Taylor, H.A., Kanarek, R.B., & Samuel, P. (2005). Effect of breakfast composition on cognitive processes in elementary school children. *Physiology & Behavior, 85*, 635–645.
14. Compart, P., & Laake, D. (2006). *Kid-friendly ADHD and autism cookbook.* Beverly, MA: Rockport Publishers.
15. Howard, A.L., Robinson, M., Smith, G. J., et al. (2012). ADHD is associated with a Western dietary pattern in adolescents. *Journal of Attention Disorders, 15*, 403-411.
16. Brown, J.F., & Lawton, M. (1986). Stress and well-being in adolescence: The moderating role of physical exercise. *Journal of Human Stress, 12*, 125-131
17. Kuo, F.E., & Taylor, A.F. (2004). A potential natural treatment for attention-deficit/hyperactivity disorder: Evidence from a national study. *American Journal of Public Health, 94*, 1580-1588.
18. Robbins, C.A., & Glasser, J.M. (2011). Using neurocognitive psychotherapy for LD and ADHD (pp 405-433) in Goldstein, S., Naglieri, J. A., & DeVries, M. (Eds). *Learning and attention disorders in adolescence and adulthood: Assessment and treatment (Second edition.)* Hoboken, NJ: Wiley.
19. Holloway, L. (1999). Holding moonbeams: Developing a group for teen girls with ADHD. *ADDvance. 2*, 12-14.
20. Babinski, D., Sibley, M., Megan, R.J., & Pelham, W. (2013). The effects of single versus mixed gender treatment for adolescent girls with ADHD. *Journal of Clinical Child and Adolescent Psychology, 41*, 243-250.
21. Chronis, A., Chacko, A., Fabiano, G., Wynbs, B., & Pelham, W. (2004). Enhancements to the behavioral parent training paradigm for families of children with ADHD: Review and future directions. *Clinical Child and Family Psychology Review, 7*, 1-27.
22. Waxmonsky, J.G., Wymbs, F.A., Pariseau, M.E., et al. (2013). A novel group therapy for children with ADHD and severe mood dysregulation. *Journal of Attention Disorders, 17*, 527-541.

23. Barkley, R.A., Edwards, G., Laneri, M., Fletcher, K., & Metevia, L. (2001). The efficacy of problem-solving communication training alone, behavior management training alone, and their combination for parent adolescent conflict in teenagers with ADHD and ODD. *Journal of Consulting and Clinical Psychology, 69*, 926-941.
24. Klingberg, T., Fernell, E., Olesen, P.J., Johnson, M., Gustafsson, P., Dahlström, K., Gillberg, C.G., Forssberg, H., & Westerberg, H. (2005). Computerized training of working memory in children with ADHD—a randomized, controlled trial. *Journal of American Academy of Child and Adolescent Psychiatry, 44*, 177-186.
25. Holmes, J., Gathercole, S.E., Place, M., Dunning, D. L., Hilton, K.A., & Elliott, J. G. (2010).Working memory deficits can be overcome: Impacts of training and medication on working memory in children with ADHD. *Applied Cognitive Psychology, 24*, 827-836.
26. Melby-Lervag, M., & Hulme, C. (2013). Is working memory training effective? A meta-analytic review. *Developmental Psychology, 49*, 270-291.
27. Zylowska, L. (2012). *The mindfulness prescription for adult ADHD*. Boston: Trumpeter Press.
28. Napoli, M., Krech, P.R., & Holley, L.C. (2005). Mindfulness training for elementary school students: The attention academy. *Journal of Applied School Psychology, 21*, 99-125.
29. British Psychological Society (BPS). (2014). Mindfulness training improves attention in children. *Science Daily, 5*. September 2014.
30. Abikoff, H., Gallagher, R., Wells, K., Murray, D., Huang, L., Lu, F., & Petkova, E. (2013). Remediating organizational functioning in children with ADHD: Immediate and long-term effects from a randomized controlled trial. *Consulting and Clinical Psychology, 81*, 113–128.
31. Biederman, J., Faraone, S. V., Mick, E., Williamson, S., Wilens, T. E., Spencer, T. J., et al. (1999). Clinical correlates of ADHD in females: Findings from a large group of girls ascertained from pediatric and psychiatric referral sources. *Journal of the American Academy of Child and Adolescent Psychiatry, 38*, 966-975.
32. Biederman, J., Petty, C.R., Monuteaux, M.C., Fried, R., Byrne, D., Mirto, T., et al. (2010). Adult psychiatric outcomes of girls with attention deficit hyperactivity disorder: 11-year follow-up in a longitudinal case-control study. *American Journal of Psychiatry, 167*, 409–417.
33. Biederman, J., Faraone, S. V., Mick, E., Williamson, S., Wilens, T. E., Spencer, T. J., et al. (1999). Clinical correlates of ADHD in females: Findings from a large group of girls ascertained from pediatric and psychiatric referral sources. *Journal of the American Academy of Child and Adolescent Psychiatry, 38*, 966-975.
34. Biederman, J., Mick, E., & Faraone, S. (1998). Depression in attention deficit hyperactivity disorder (ADHD) children: "True" depression or demoralization? *Journal of Affective Disorders, 47*, 113-122.
35. Marks, A., Nichols, M., Blasey, C., Kato, P., & Huffman, L. (2002). Girls with ADHD and associated behavioral problems: Patterns of comorbidity. *North American Journal of Psychology, 4*, -.
36. Levy F., Hay, D.A., Bennett, K.S., & McStephen, M. (2005). Gender differences in ADHD subtype comorbidity. *Journal of the American Academy of Child and Adolescent Psychiatry, 44*, 368-376.
37. Biederman, J., Petty, C.R., & Monuteaux, M.C., et al. (2008). The longitudinal course comorbid oppositional defiant disorder in girls with attention-deficit/hyperactivity disorder: Findings from a controlled 5-year prospective longitudinal follow-up study. *Journal of Developmental and Behavioral Pediatrics, 29*, 501-507.
38. Biederman J, Faraone S, Milberger S, et al. (1996). Predictors of persistence and remission of ADHD into adolescence: Results from a four-year prospective follow-up study. *Journal of the American Academy of Child and Adolescent Psychiatry, 35*, 343-351.

39. Burke, J., Hipwell, A., & Loeber, R. (2010). Dimensions of oppositional defiant disorder as predictors of depression and conduct disorder in preadolescent girls. *Journal of the American Academy of Child and Adolescent Psychiatry, 49*, 484-492.
40. Stepp, S., Burke, J., Hipwell, A., & Loeber, R. (2012). Trajectories of attention deficit hyperactivity disorder and oppositional defiant disorder symptoms as precursors of borderline personality disorder symptoms in adolescent girls. *Journal of Abnormal Child Psychology, 40*, 7-20.
41. Horner, B.R., & Scheibe, K.E. (1997). Prevalence and implications of attention-deficit hyperactivity disorder among adolescents in treatment for substance abuse. *Journal of the American Academy of Child and Adolescent Psychiatry, 36*, 30-36.
42. Stulz, N., Hepp, U., Gachter, C., Martin-Soelch, C., Spindler, A., & Milos, G. (2013). The severity of ADHD and eating disorder symptoms: A correlational study. *BMC Psychiatry, 13*, 44.
43. Erhart, M., Herpertz-Dahlmann, B., et al. (2012). Examining the relationships between attention-deficit/hyperactivity disorder and overweight in children and adolescents. *European Child and Adolescent Psychiatry, 21*, 39-49.
44. Owens, J. (2008). A clinical overview of sleep and attention-deficit/hyperactivity disorder in children and adolescents. *Journal of the Canadian Academy of Child and Adolescent Psychiatry, 18*, 92-102.
45. Mitchell, M.D., Gehrman, P., Perlis, M., & Umscheld, C. (2012). Comparative effectiveness of cognitive behavioral therapy for insomnia: A systematic review. *Disorders of Sleep, 12*, 80-89.

CHAPTER ELEVEN

1. Biederman, J., Spencer, T., & Wilens, T. (2004). Evidence-based pharmacotherapy for attention-deficit hyperactivity disorder. *International Journal of Neuropcychopharmacology, 7*, 77-97.
2. Jensen, P.S., Hinshaw, S.P., Swanson, J.M., Greenhill, L.L., Conners, C.K., et al. (2001). Findings from the NIMH multimodal treatment study of ADHD (MTA): Implications and applications for primary care providers. *Journal of Developmental and Behavioral Pediatrics, 22*, 60-73.
3. Greenhill, L.L. (2002). Stimulant medication treatment of children with attention-deficit/hyperactivity disorder. In: *Attention deficit hyperactivity disorder: State of science. Best practices*, Jensen, P.S., Cooper, J.R. (eds). Kingston, NJ: Civic Research Institute.
4. Frankel, F.F., Cantwell, D., Myatt, R., & Feinberg, D.T. (1999). Do stimulants improve self-esteem in children with ADHD and peer problems? *Journal of Child and Adolescent Psychopharmacology, 9*, 185-194.
5. Karpenko, V., Owens, J.S., Evangelista, N.M., & Dodds, C. (2009). Clinically significant symptom change in children with ADHD: Does it correspond with reliable improvement in functioning? *Journal of Clinical Psychology, 65*, 76-93.
6. American Academy of Pediatrics. (2011). ADHD: Clinical practice guideline for the diagnosis, evaluation, and treatment of attention-deficit/hyperactivity disorder in children and adolescents, *Pediatrics, 128*, 1016-1018.
7. American Academy of Child and Adolescent Psychiatry. (2007). Practice parameter for the assessment and treatment of children and adolescents with attention-deficit/hyperactivity disorder. *Journal of the American Academy of Child and Adolescent Psychiatry, 46*, 904-906.
8. American Academy of Pediatrics. (2011). ADHD: Clinical practice guideline for the diagnosis, evaluation, and treatment of attention-deficit/hyperactivity disorder in children and adolescents, *Pediatrics, 128*, 1016-1018.
9. Steven, Pliszka, AACAP Work Group on Quality Issues. (2007). Practice parameter for the assessment and treatment of children and adolescents with attention-deficit/hyperactivity disorder. *Journal of the American Academy of Child and Adolescent Psychiatry, 47*, 894-904.

10. Sharp, W.S., Walter, J.M., Marsh, W.L., Ritchie, G.F., Hamburger, S.D., & Castellanos, F.X. (1999). ADHD in girls: Clinical comparability of a research sample. *Journal of the American Academy of Child and Adolescent Psychiatry, 38*, 40-47.
11. Lee, L., Kepple, J., Wang, Y., Freestonem S., Bakhtiar, R., Wang, Y., & Hossain, M. (2003). Bioavailability of modified-release methylphenidate: Influence of high-fat breakfast when administered intact and when capsule content sprinkled on applesauce. *Biopharmaceutics and Drug Disposition, 24*, 233-243.
12. McGough, J.J., Wigal, S.B., Abikoff, H., Turnbow, J.M., Posner, K., & Moon, E. (2006). A randomized, double-blind, placebo controlled, laboratory classroom assessment of methylphenidate transdermal system in children with ADHD. *Journal of Attention Disorders, 9*, 476-485.
13. Findling, R., & Lopez, F.A. (2005). The effects of transdermal methylphenidate with reference to Concerta in ADHD. *Scientific Proceedings of the American Academy of Child and Adolescent Psychiatry, 32*, 123.
14. Findling, R.L., Bukstein, O.G., Melmed, R.D., et al. (2008). A randomized, double-blind, placebo controlled, parallel-group study of methylphenidate transdermal system in pediatric patients with attention-deficit/hyperactivity disorder. *Journal of Clinical Psychiatry, 69*, 149-159.
15. Findling, R.L., Bukstein, O.G., Melmed, R.D., López, F.A., Sallee, F.R., Arnold, L.E., & Pratt, R.D. (2008). A randomized, double-blind, placebo-controlled, parallel-group study of methylphenidate transdermal system in pediatric patients with attention-deficit/hyperactivity disorder. *Journal of Clinical Psychiatry, 69*, 149-159.
16. Adesman, A.R. (2001). The diagnosis and management of attention-deficit/hyperactivity disorder in pediatric patients. *Primary Care Companion Journal of Clinical Psychiatry, 3*, 66-77.
17. Cyr, M., & Brown, C.S. (1998). Current drug therapy recommendations for the treatment of attention deficit hyperactivity disorder. *Drugs, 56*, 215-223.
18. Corkum, P., Panton, R., Ironside, S., MacPherson, M., & Williams, T. (2007). Acute impact of immediate release methyphenidate administered three times a day on sleep in children with attention-deficit/hyperactivity disorder. *Journal of Pediatric Psychology, 33*, 368-379.
19. McGough, J.J., Biederman, J., Wigal, S.B., Lopez, F.A., McCracken, J.T., et al. (2005). Long term tolerability and effectiveness of once-daily mixed amphetamine salts (Adderall XR) in children with ADHD. *Journal of the Academy of Child and Adolescent Psychiatry, 44*, 530-538.
20. Wolraich, M.L., Greenhill, L.L., Pelham, W., Swanson, J., Wilens, T., Palumbom D., Atkins, M., McBurnett, K., Bukstein, O., & August. G. (2001). Randomized, controlled trial of oros-methylphenidate once a day in children with attention-deficit/hyperactivity disorder. *Pediatrics, 108*, 883-892.
21. Biederman, J., Krishnan, S., Zhang, Y., McGough, J.J., & Findling, R.L. (2007). Efficacy and tolerability of lisdexamfetamine dimesylate (NRP-104) in children with attention-deficit/hyperactivity disorder: A phase III, multicenter, randomized, double-blind, forced-dose, parallel-group study. *Clinical Therapeutics, 29*, 450-463.
22. Swanson, J., Elliott, G.R., Greenhill, L.L., et al. (2007). Effects of stimulant medication on growth rates across three years of the MTA follow-up. *Journal of the Academy of Child and Adolescent Psychiatry, 46*, 1015-1027.
23. American Academy of Child and Adolescent Psychiatry. (2007). Practice parameter for the assessment and treatment of children and adolescents with attention-deficit/hyperactivity disorder. *Journal of the American Academy of Child and Adolescent Psychiatry, 46*, 904-906.
24. Berridge, C.W., & Devilbiss, D.M. (2011). Psychostimulants as cognitive enhancers: The prefrontal cortex, catecholamines, and attention-deficit/hyperactivity disorder. *Biological Psychiatry, 69*, e101-111.

25. Volkow, N.D., Fowler, J.S., Wang, G., Ding, Y., & Gatley, S.J. (2002). Mechanism of action of methylphenidate: Insights from PET imaging studies. *Journal of Attention Disorders, 6*, Suppl 1, S31-44.
26. Schweitzer, J.B., Lee, D.O., Hanford, R.B., Tagamets, M.A., Hoffman, J.M., Grafton, S.T., & Kilts, C.D. (2003). A positron emission tomography study of methylphenidate in adults with ADHD: Alterations in resting blood flow and predicting treatment response. *Neuropsychopharmacology, 28*, 967-973.
27. Spencer, R.C., Klein, R.M., & Berridge, C.W. (2012). Psychostimulants act within the prefrontal cortex to improve cognitive function. *Biological Psychiatry, 72*, 221-227.
28. Gamo, N.J., Wang, M., & Arnsten, A.F. (2010). Methylphenidate and atomoxetine enhance prefrontal function through 2-adrenergic and dopamine D1 receptors. *Journal of the American Academy of Child and Adolescent Psychiatry, 49*, 1011-1023.
29. Schmeichel, B.E., & Berridge, C.W. (2013). Neurocircuitry underlying the preferential sensitivity of prefrontal catecholamines to low-dose psychostimulants. *Neuropsychopharmacology, 38*, 1078-1084.
30. Connor, D.F., Fletcher, K.E., & Swanson, J.M. (1999). A meta-analysis of clonidine for symptoms of attention-deficit hyperactivity disorder. *Journal of the American Academy of Child and Adolescent Psychiatry, 38*, 1551-1559.
31. Sharp, W.S., Walter, J.M., Marsh, W.L., Ritchie, G.F., Hamburger, S.D., & Castellanos, F.X. (1999). ADHD in girls: Clinical comparability of a research sample. *Journal of the American Academy of Child and Adolescent Psychiatry, 38*, 40-47.
32. Safer, D.J., & Malever, M. (2000). Stimulant treatment in Maryland public schools. *Pediatrics, 106*, 533-539.
33. Wolraich, ML. Recognizing, understanding and treating co-occurring conditions. Poster presented at the 16th Annual International Conference of Children and Adults with Attention-Deficit/Hyperactivity Disorder (CHADD). October 2004.
34. Biederman, J., Wigal, S.B., Spencer, T.J., McGough, J.J., & Mays, D.A. (2006). A post hoc subgroup analysis of an 18-day randomized controlled trial comparing the tolerability and efficacy of mixed amphetamine salts extended release and atomoxetine in school-age girls with attention-deficit/hyperactivity disorder. *Clinical Therapeutics, 28*, 280-293.
35. Barbaresi, W.J., Katusic, S.K., Colligan, R.C., Weaver, A.L., Leibson, C.L., & Jacobsen, S.J (2006). Long-term stimulant medication treatment of attention-deficit/hyperactivity disorder: Results from a population-based study. *Journal of Developmental and Behavioral Pediatrics, 27*, 1-10.
36. Mikami, A.Y., Cox, D.J., Davis, M.T., Wilson, H.K., Merkel, R.L., & Burket, R. (2009). Sex differences in effectiveness of extended-release stimulant medication among adolescents with attention-deficit/hyperactivity disorder. *Journal of Clinical Psychology in Medical Settings, 16*, 233-242.
37. West, S.A., Muniz, R., Quinn, P., Wigal, S., Pestreich, L., & Wang, J. (2004). The GRACE study: An evaluation of girls, Ritalin, and ADHD. Poster presented at the 51st Annual Meeting of the American Academy of Child and Adolescent Psychiatry, October 19-24, Washington, DC.
38. Biederman, J., Wigal, S.B., Spencer, T.J., McGough, J.J., & Mays, D.A. (2006). A post hoc subgroup analysis of an 18-day randomized controlled trial comparing the tolerability and efficacy of mixed amphetamine salts extended release and atomoxetine in school-age girls with attention-deficit/hyperactivity disorder. *Clinical Therapeutics, 28*, 280-293.
39. Greenhill, L.L., Abikoff, H.B., Arnold, L.E., et al. (1996). Medication treatment strategies in the MTA study: Relevance to clinicians and researchers. *Journal of the American Academy of Child and Adolescent Psychiatry, 35*, 1304-1.

40. American Academy of Pediatrics. (2011). ADHD: Clinical practice guideline for the diagnosis, evaluation, and treatment of attention-deficit/hyperactivity disorder in children and adolescents, *Pediatrics, 128*, 1016-1018.
41. Connor, D.F. (2002). Preschool attention deficit hyperactivity disorder: A review of prevalence, diagnosis, neurobiology, and stimulant treatment. *Journal of Developmental and Behavioral Pediatrics, 23*, 1-9.
42. Wigal, T., Greenhill, L., Chuang. S., McGough, J., Vitiello, B., et al. (2006). Safety and tolerability of methylphenidate in preschool children with ADHD. *Journal of the American Academy of Child and Adolescent Psychiatry, 45*, 1294-1303.
43. Greenhill, L., Kollins, S., Abikoff, H., McCracken, J., Riddle, M., et al. (2006). Efficacy and safety of immediate-release methylphenidate treatment for preschoolers with ADHD. *Journal of the American Academy of Child and Adolescent Psychiatry, 45*, 1284-1293.
44. Wigal, T., Greenhill, L., Chuang. S., McGough, J., Vitiello, B., et al. (2006). Safety and tolerability of methylphenidate in preschool children with ADHD. *Journal of the American Academy of Child and Adolescent Psychiatry, 45*, 1294-1303.
45. Biederman, J., Mick, E., & Faraone, S. (1998). Depression in attention deficit hyperactivity disorder (ADHD) children: "True" depression or demoralization? *Journal of Affective Disorders, 47*, 113-122.
46. American Academy of Child and Adolescent Psychiatry. (2007). Practice parameter for the assessment and treatment of children and adolescents with attention-deficit/hyperactivity disorder. *Journal of the American Academy of Child and Adolescent Psychiatry, 46*, 904-906.
47. Biederman, J., Faraone, S. V., Mick, E., Williamson, S., Wilens, T. E., Spencer, T. J., et al. (1999). Clinical correlates of ADHD in females: Findings from a large group of girls ascertained from pediatric and psychiatric referral sources. *Journal of the American Academy of Child and Adolescent Psychiatry, 38*, 966-975.
48. Biederman, J., Petty, C.R., Monuteaux, M.C., Fried, R., Byrne, D., Mirto, T., et al. (2010). Adult psychiatric outcomes of girls with attention deficit hyperactivity disorder: 11-year follow-up in a longitudinal case-control study. *American Journal of Psychiatry, 167*, 409–417.
49. American Academy of Child and Adolescent Psychiatry. (2007). Practice parameter for the assessment and treatment of children and adolescents with attention-deficit/hyperactivity disorder. *Journal of the American Academy of Child and Adolescent Psychiatry, 46*, 904-906.
50. American Academy of Child and Adolescent Psychiatry. (2007). Practice parameter for the assessment and treatment of children and adolescents with attention-deficit/hyperactivity disorder. *Journal of the American Academy of Child and Adolescent Psychiatry, 46*, 904-906.
51. Gammon, G.D., & Brown, T.E. (1993). Fluoxetine and methylphenidate in combination for treatment of attention deficit disorder and comorbid depressive disorder. *Journal of Child and Adolescent Psychopharmacology, 3*, 1-10.
52. Findling, R.L. (1996). Open-label treatment of comorbid depression and attentional disorders with co-administration of serotonin reuptake inhibitors and psychostimulants in children, adolescents, and adults: A case series. *Journal of Child and Adolescent Psychopharmacology, 6*, 165-75.
53. Gallanter, C., & Liebenluft, E. (2008). Frontiers between attention deficit hyperactivity disorder and bipolar disorder. *Child and Adolescent Psychiatric Clinics of North America, 17*, -246, viii-ix.
54. Giedd, J.N. (2000). Bipolar disorder and attention-deficit/hyperactivity disorder in children and adolescents. *Journal of Clinical Psychiatry, 6*, 31-34.
55. Mikami, A.Y., Hinshaw, S.P., Patterson, K.A., & Lee, J.C. (2008). Eating pathology among adolescent girls with attention-deficit/hyperactivity disorder. *Journal of Abnormal Psychology, 117*, 225–235.

56. Fliers, E.A., Buitelaar, J.K., Maras, A., Bul, K., Höhle, E., Faraone, S.V., Franke, B., & Rommelse, N.N. (2013). ADHD is a risk factor for overweight and obesity in children. *Journal of Developmental and Behavioral Pediatrics, 34*, 566-574.
57. Agranat-Meged, A.N., Deitcher, C., Goldzweig, G., Leibenson, L., Stein, M., & Galili-Weisstub, E. (2005). Childhood obesity and attention deficit/hyperactivity disorder: A newly described comorbidity in obese hospitalized children. *International Journal of Eating Disorders, 37*, 357-359.
58. Kim, J., Mutyala, B., Agiovlasitis, S., & Fernhall, B. (2011). Health behaviors and obesity among US children with attention deficit hyperactivity disorder by gender and medication use. *Preventative Medicine, 52*, 218-222.
59. Dukarm, C. (2005). Bulimia nervosa and ADD: A possible role for stimulant medication. *Journal of Women's Health, 14*, 345–350.
60. Dukarm, C. (2006). *Pieces of a Puzzle: The link between eating disorders and ADHD*. Washington, DC: Advantage Books.
61. Bhatia, S.C., & Bhatia, S.K. (2002). Diagnosis and treatment of premenstrual dysphoric disorder. *American Family Physician, 66*, 1239-1248.
62. Steiner, M., Pearlstein, T., Cohen, L.S., Endicott, J., Kornstein, S.G., Roberts, C., Roberts, D.L., & Yonkers, K. (2006). Expert guidelines for the treatment of severe PMS, PMDD, and comorbidities: The role of SSRIs. *Journal of Women's Health, 15*, 57-69.

CHAPTER TWELVE

1. American Psychiatric Association. (2000). *Diagnostic and statistical manual of mental disorders, Fourth Edition*. Arlington, VA: American Psychiatric Publishers.
2. American Psychiatric Association. (2013). *Diagnostic and statistical manual of mental disorders, Fifth edition*. Arlington, VA: American Psychiatric Publishers.

INDEX

B

F

G

H

I

K

L

M

N

O

S